Life on An Alien Planet

A journey through school for a young boy with
Asperger's and Pathological Demand Avoidance
Syndrome

Katie Stott

This book would not have been possible without support from the people around me.

To my wonderful husband he made sense of everything for me. They sure do say that relationships are hard work and ours has withstood through thick and thin. We worked as a team, without us working as a team I don't think we would have achieved everything we did for our son.

Tyler – My eldest son, you're growing up now and approaching your 18th birthday. You are a caring young man who I am very proud of.

My mum for just being there to listen to me on the other end of the phone. All you need is an ear sometimes. My mum has had unconditional patience with Fraser. Sometimes the way Fraser would use his words so literally would hurt her feelings, but she's learnt to take things with a pinch of salt as we all have.

Ruth and Sarah - My lovely friends who have been there since day one when I needed support and help on the whole system. They have bent over backwards, listened to my worries and have given me some wonderful words of wisdom.

Yvonne Newbold – Who taught me a completely different way to parent. She opened my eyes and talked a lot of sense. She's an inspiration fighting her own battles and helping others.

Zoe – My playground mum back in mainstream. She opened my eyes right at the beginning and encouraged me to push for the support we needed. She stood in the playground with me - heard my worries, saw my tears. She made the journey walking through the school gates a little easier every day.

Contents

Introduction

3rd September 2016

Opening the bedroom curtains that morning, I was greeted by a mild autumn day with the onset of winter seemingly still far away. There was excited anticipation in the house as our four-year-old son, Fraser, put on his crisp grey and blue primary school uniform for the first time. Not only two minutes ago had it seemed we were leaving the hospital after his birth and before we knew it, he was taking his first tentative steps into a new form of independence.

My husband, Nigel, had taken the morning off work and fussed over Fraser to make sure that his uniform sat correctly before checking we had everything for the umpteenth time. We drove the short journey to school with the same thoughts any parent taking their child to school for the first time would have. We hoped he quickly made friends, enjoyed the meals, excelled academically and fitted in with the rest of the class.

Near the school, we parked up at the side of a leafy suburban road. Fraser stepped out of the car and clasped Nigel's hand as he boldly walked towards the school. This was a new chapter in his life and looking down at this small boy, just four years old, I was nervous but also excited for him. We had done everything we could to secure him a place at the best school in the area. As we walked up the street, the school came into sight and we crossed the road to make our way through the main entrance. As we left him with his new class that day little could we have known what was to come.

Within a few months, Fraser was smashing up school property, lashing out at teachers and classmates and was being restrained by teachers on a regular basis. Over time he became ostracised from his classmates and spent hours alone at a desk outside the classroom or in the headteacher's office. We had no idea what had suddenly got into our beautiful little boy. Life at home was a little better but we still experienced sudden outbursts of anger that we had never experienced before. The simplest of things – telling Fraser that we were all going out to the shops or that we had to change our plans due to wet weather would instil a rage within him.

To be frank, the school had no idea what to do with him either. He was attending a Catholic school that had never seen behaviour of this sort. The various specialists that attended school recommended strategies that didn't work, and we began to get desperate. Over time, Fraser received a diagnosis of Asperger syndrome which is part of the autistic spectrum, but that still didn't provide the answer we were looking for. Autism strategies were employed to little or no effect on his behaviour.

That's when we discovered that Fraser had a condition known as Pathological Demand Avoidance

(PDA) which can be found in a small percentage of children with an autism spectrum disorder.

What we cover in this book

In this book, we detail our experiences of home, school and our journey to a better place. Parents of children with special educational needs (SEN) will no doubt identify with the struggle and the emotions we went through as parents when dealing with the constant churn of issues at school and trying to make progress with the local authority for an Education, Health and Care Plan (EHCP). In the United Kingdom, a child with special needs will need an EHCP to gain access to a specialist setting (i.e. specialist school) and resources that will help them thrive in their education. However, getting an EHCP is no easy feat for a number of reasons. It is likely many mainstream schools may have never gone through the process to obtain an EHCP for a child. Even if your child is having issues at school, the headteacher or SENCO (Special Educational Needs Co-Ordinator) through lack of experience or knowledge may believe that your child does not meet the criteria for an EHCP.

Never take what you are told for granted. We were told that our child would never obtain an EHCP as he wasn't "non-verbal autistic". A few months later, he was finally given an EHCP. This doesn't mean we had an easy ride to get one, we didn't - but if we had believed everything we were told we wouldn't have got the support our child now has. An EHCP is a legal document. Local Authorities will not dish them out easily and many parents face a fight to get one for their child.

For the majority of parents, this will be the first and only time they go through the process of getting their child the support they need. Every situation will be different, and each local authority will have a slightly different way of doing things. However, I firmly believe that we ultimately achieved our goal because we spent many long hours educating ourselves on the law, going through the fine detail of any document that was sent to us and not being afraid to stand our ground and fight for what we believed in. Nothing good comes without hard work and I believe our efforts reaped the best result.

Once we obtained an EHCP for our son, we then had another fight to ensure he could attend a specialist school that could cater to his needs. The LA was keen to place him in a local specialist school that would cost less for them but would not necessarily meet all his needs. Our story details how we found the right school for our son in a neighbouring authority that would ultimately cost the LA a good deal more. Through approaching things in the right way we managed to secure the school placement we desired.

Fraser is now a happy child who thrives albeit with the odd challenge here and there.

We hope that this book helps parents in a similar situation to us. There was no "map" to show us what we needed to do - how to turn around the unhappy situation we were in and to make things better. Looking back on the early days, it does feel like Fraser's situation wasn't taken as seriously as it should have been. We didn't know any better and it was only through the power of the internet and tapping into specialist organisations did we get more clued up. We cannot overemphasise the help that Facebook groups gave us, though they can be a double-edged sword with a lot of hearsay and inaccuracy floating around. Always check your facts before relying on information on social media. Organisations such as IPSEA (www.ipsea.org.uk), run training courses on special needs law which we attended and websites such as Special Needs Jungle (www.specialneedsjungle.com) were an invaluable resource.

When the trouble at school started and they realised that Fraser might need specialist help the number of acronyms that were thrown around was mind-boggling. We do detail the acronyms at the end of the book to help with this. We use a lot of acronyms in this book but only after we have explained what they mean in some detail.

What is Pathological Demand Avoidance?

Throughout this book, we refer a lot to Pathological Demand Avoidance (PDA). Fraser was initially diagnosed with Asperger syndrome which is an Autism spectrum disorder (ASD). It was only later when ASD strategies weren't working that he was finally diagnosed with PDA (which is now believed to be part of ASD).

Pathological Demand Avoidance (PDA) is a relatively uncommon condition. Those experiencing PDA will have an overwhelming need to resist or avoid perceived demands. The word "perceived", in our opinion, is quite important here. If you were speaking to a person with PDA and used a certain tone or phrase to make a request, then it may be perceived by the person with PDA that you were making a demand of them and they would respond as such. This is even if there was no intention in the delivery of the statement to make a demand. However, a different tone of voice may elicit a different response. It is our experience that a more passive tone of voice works better with our son.

The avoidance of demands stems from a need to be in control believed to be driven by anxiety. Individuals with a demand avoidant profile may appear on the surface to have a typical level of social understanding and communication skills. Whilst they can use these skills to manipulate a situation the actual social awareness and comprehension they have isn't all it seems.

There are typical characteristics displayed by those who suffer from PDA. These include:

An obsessive resistance to everyday demands and requests

Everyday requests, such as announcing we were going to the shops, visiting family or changing where we were going on a planned outing could induce a severe change in mood and behaviour in Fraser. He would shout, lash out at us and do anything to avoid the "demand" that was being made on him.

This is typical behaviour of a PDA child and was a shock when it first started happening to us. The behaviour started at school, so not knowing that our son had PDA at that stage, we believed his issues were associated with the school environment.

However, when the behaviour also started at home, we knew something else was driving this sudden change.

PDA children, due to their age, are naturally spontaneous in their reaction to demands and their behaviours will normally be restricted to physical outbursts. However, as children get older, the way they avoid demands can become more complex. For example, they may try to distract the person making the demand or try and negotiate with them

In some cases, children may withdraw into fantasy but this is not something we have personally seen in our son. What is particularly interesting with PDA children is that they may adopt different avoidance strategies depending on who is making the demand on them. This demonstrates a level of social understanding that is enough to manipulate the person making the demand but if they still fail to avoid the demand this can quickly disintegrate into a meltdown – punching, shouting and throwing objects. Many a time we remember a projectile hitting the windscreen from the back seat of the car when things weren't going well!

Can appear to be sociable but lack understanding of social norms

People with PDA may appear like everyone else on the surface but may exhibit social behaviours that are viewed as odd by other people.

A few examples of typical behaviours include:

- Use of manipulative or outrageous behaviour

in social settings to avoid demands
- Sudden changes in mood that can be associated with a need to control
- 'Surface' sociability, reflected in social peculiarity, difficulties with peers and lack of social constraint
- Comfortable in role play and pretending.

In children with PDA, you can see how this may become even more extreme. Sometimes the apparent need for a PDA child to be in control can be overwhelming for those around them. It should be remembered that although it may appear that the child is seeking to dominate, they are actually trying to minimise uncertainty to limit their anxiety.

Excessive mood swings and acts on impulse

While many people on the autistic spectrum can have problems regulating their emotions, it has been found that this trait is often emphasised in those with a demand avoidant profile. The speed at which they can change their mood is like a power switch going on and off.

For the casual observer, the emotions can seem overly dramatic and often with no obvious trigger. However, these moods happen in PDA children due to a perceived pressure or demand and their apparent need to be in control.

When Fraser attended children's parties, he could quickly go from having a good time to an extreme meltdown. The severity of these mood swings did seem dramatic but quite often, he would quickly be over them and keen to join the party again.

Severe behavioural issues

As discussed in the previous sections, mood swings can trigger in an instant. This can also be combined with a tendency for people with a demand avoidant profile to be unable to regulate emotions such as anger. In essence, the behaviour that arises is often due to extreme anxiety or panic attacks and strategies of reassurance and de-escalation should be adopted.

When Fraser exhibits extreme behaviour or anger we always speak to him calmly and give him space which de-escalates the situation. It should be remembered that the behaviour of a person with a demand avoidant profile will differ in various settings. For Fraser, he was particularly anxious at school where he had less control over his environment. Ultimately, this led to exclusion from school for him and a period of home-schooling.

Is PDA a recognised condition?

At the time of writing, PDA is not currently included in either of the autism diagnostic manuals (DSM-V and ICD-10). The validity of this profile as part of ASD remains a contentious subject among many professionals. For this reason, we struggled when trying to encourage the LA and school to change their strategies when dealing with Fraser. Many standard ASD strategies were deployed, which in our view, did not work for our son. However, much effort is going into making PDA a recognised condition. For example, the PDA Society (**www.pdasociety.org.uk**) are doing fantastic work to increase recognition and understanding of the condition. Their website provides a detailed resource for parents, carers, teachers and professionals.

Chapter 1 - A New Beginning

June 2008

My life in 2008 felt like it was finally clicking into place. I had recently divorced after eight years of marriage and was now a single twenty-eight-year-old mum with a six-year-old child. Nigel had stepped into my life in May 2008 and we had a whirlwind romance. We clicked immediately upon meeting and Nigel, also recently divorced, seemed unphased about taking on me and my son. Two weeks after meeting he had moved into my home and just five months after that, we bought our first house together in the beautiful city of York, where I had lived all my life.

We had a good year of getting used to family life together - Nigel was leaving behind a ten-year marriage but had no children, so things were slightly different for him. During this year he was adapting and taking on the role of stepdad to my son Tyler, but everything was coming together.

Nigel and I were deeply in love and there was nothing more we wanted than to have our own child. We both felt that there would never be a "right time" and we started planning immediately. Say what you like about us, we didn't like to wait for anything! I think that's just the way things go for us, even now things never seem to slow down. We make a lot of decisions together and then work as a team to see them through. Taking action is so important as it is the only way anything can get done.

Around this time, we agreed we should book our first holiday together before we had a new addition to the family that would require our attention for the next eighteen years. Never one to shy away from an adventure, we pored over the brochures and opted for a week in the party capital of Las Vegas followed by a more relaxed week in the small town of Clearwater, Florida. This was the holiday of a lifetime for me. I had never been further than Spain before and the thought of a holiday in the USA made me so excited.

I remember so clearly being sat on the plane, high above the clouds, feeling like I was literally on my own cloud nine. I also remember wondering whether I might already be pregnant? If I was, it felt different from before, I had different symptoms. I didn't feel sick, but my breasts were sore. Deep down I had that feeling but then I thought I couldn't be, we had only just started talking about trying for a baby a month ago, things surely couldn't move that fast? I then started to panic thinking about being in Vegas, I wouldn't be able to drink alcohol, so I would need to find out sooner than later. As the plane started to descend into Las Vegas we caught sight of a powerful light shining up into the night sky like a beacon. The beam came from our hotel, the Luxor, that would be our home for the next seven days and the place where our lives changed forever. As the plane wheels touched the tarmac my thoughts were already on planning what we needed to do. As soon as we stepped out of the airport and into a taxi, finding a pharmacy so that we could buy a pregnancy test was the main priority on my mind.

The taxi cruised down the Las Vegas strip where the bright lights shining from the hotels and casinos overwhelm the senses. I had been looking forward to this and my mind was temporarily distracted as we pulled up to the main doors of the famous pyramid-shaped Luxor hotel. We hauled our bags up to reception, marvelling at the immensity of the main reception area, that was adorned in fake Egyptian relics and towering Sphinx. We managed to check-in quickly and headed up to our room in order to dump our bags before heading into a warm and busy Nevada evening. It didn't take long to find a pharmacy and clutching a pregnancy test we headed back to the room in anticipation.

We sat on the bed, whilst the test sat on the sink in the bathroom, waiting for the required number of minutes to pass. As soon as the time was up, we burst back into the bathroom to check. "Oh my god", I said excitedly "The line is there … it's positive!". I couldn't contain my excitement and we started jumping up and down like madmen right there in that Vegas hotel room. But wait. What if the test was faulty? I was suddenly worried that the test might be showing a false result.

In the end, we purchased three pregnancy tests. Yes, I know. It took me three tests to believe that I was actually pregnant. I couldn't believe it had happened so quick. We were delighted. Our holiday in Vegas wasn't quite the trip we had planned. Wild nights were exchanged for hot chocolate and bed for 9pm most nights, but we didn't care. We were away together, having fun and exploring with one very special baby inside me.

My pregnancy felt very different this time around. I had no sickness and actually enjoyed the feeling of being pregnant. We decided to have a private 3D baby scan that would reveal the sex of the baby a little earlier than the NHS scan. The baby's hands covered everything up to begin with and it took three attempts before we found out … we were having a boy!

The rest of the pregnancy was completely normal – no dramas or worries and I was booked in to have a C-section on the 23rd June 2010. I remember nervously waiting with Nigel, sat in the hospital corridor contemplating how in just a few hours, our lives would change forever. It wasn't long before a nurse popped her head around the corner and called us through to the preparation room. The nurse asked me to change into a hospital gown and then indicated I should sit on the edge of the operating theatre table. I sat down with my lower back exposed as the anaesthetist administered the epidural into my back. Whilst this was happening, Nigel was shown to a small room to change into a surgeon's gown (luckily, he wasn't delivering the baby). We were called through into the delivery room and all I remember after a few minutes were the first cries of my gorgeous baby boy.

Fraser was born into this world at 10.25am and little did we know how our lives would change forever.

I was moved to a bed in a quiet room next to the delivery room where I was given my freshly cleaned up and now very calm gorgeous boy. He was a beautiful baby just as I imagined, he inherited the olive looking skin that his daddy had with beautiful big brown eyes. We were in love. After cuddling my boy for a few minutes, I passed him over to his daddy. I'm not sure how he managed it but Nigel, who had never held a baby in his life, somehow managed to let Fraser slip through his arms. Despite the soft landing back on the bed Fraser was heading for, the panic on Nigel's face quickly turned to relief as he managed to catch his baby boy and we all broke into giggles at something only a new dad could do! This was going to be a steep learning curve for Nigel but I could tell he was already in love with his son and it made me so excited inside to realise that we finally had our boy and everything was going to be perfect.

I stayed in the hospital for about 48 hours before they let us go home. Nigel arrived with the car seat we had spent hours shopping for a few months earlier and Fraser seemed so tiny when he was sat in it. I had never seen Nigel drive more carefully as we drove the short distance home.

I was eager to breastfeed Fraser as my previous time with Tyler did not go well. When I gave birth to Tyler in 2001, I was only 21 and I felt that I had given up on trying to breastfeed too quickly. With a more mature head on my shoulders this time I was determined that I would make it work. However, no matter how hard I tried it just wasn't working. I clearly remember the tears of frustration running down my face as time after time Fraser just didn't seem interested. I tried and tried until the midwife told me that we needed to get our baby some milk from a bottle before we were admitted back into the hospital. I was heartbroken but at the same time relieved that Fraser was getting the milk he needed and hopefully he would feel more settled.

Over the next few months, I had a baby that never seemed happy. He wouldn't go to sleep very easily, and he didn't seem to be developing a sleeping pattern. Like all parents, we knew this was part of having a baby but intuitively something didn't feel right at the same time. I do wonder if the disruption and upset in the early months was due to the unique sensory profile that he carries around with him to this day? We questioned the community nurse, followed all the advice available about colic and nothing was working. As a very tired and concerned mother, I was back at the GP's surgery seeking answers before long. I was worried, Fraser wasn't just a crying child, there must be something else wrong that hadn't yet been identified. Our GP carried out further tests and eventually discovered a potential milk allergy. This news actually came as a relief, we could put Fraser's unrest down to the allergy which we were assured he would grow out of. We followed the advice from our GP and from that day onwards Fraser was on prescribed milk from the chemist.

The rest of Fraser's years as a baby were nothing unusual but certain things do resonate with me when I look back. Restaurants were a nightmare, he definitely wouldn't sit calmly in his high seat and we always seemed to come out of the restaurant covered in more food than we had actually eaten.

When I had Tyler at 21 years old, I have to be honest and say that my parents played a huge part in bringing him up whilst I went out to work. For this reason, I missed out on his baby stages, so this time around I wanted to bring my baby up, raise him myself and cherish every step of motherhood. I was lucky to be able to stay at home this time around too. We were in a position where Nigel earned enough for us to do this. I was looking forward to when Fraser could start a playgroup and I could watch him grow and develop in this world up until he was ready to start school.

Playgroup went well, I didn't really notice anything peculiar back then. The staff did comment on how Fraser wouldn't really interact much with the other children and they tried to help him develop his social skills. He just didn't seem interested though. The puzzle table was a firm favourite of his and so was anything that involved building. His dad bought him a big box of building blocks and they would play with these together - building houses, towers and walls. He didn't get involved in much imaginative play but he would love inventing and creating things.

What really struck us about Fraser during his toddler years was his quirky sense of humour and his unabashed nature. He seemed oblivious to other's thoughts and opinions and wouldn't hesitate to get up and dance at the kids disco on holiday in Spain or jump off his chair in the middle of a restaurant and bust his moves when a song he liked came on. He truly danced like no-one was watching. Even to this day, he doesn't seem to care about other's thoughts and opinions, and this continues to be one of his best and strongest attributes.

I did notice that when we did song time at playgroup, he was probably the only child that wanted to shoot out of my lap and sit on his own at the other side of the church hall. Whilst leaving

Fraser on his own at playgroup wasn't a problem in itself, when I collected him it didn't seem like he had enjoyed himself. I stayed and watched a few times and he didn't want to join in with the other children - the fascination of the bricks or building something kept him amused. Nigel was working in Leeds, so we moved from York over to Leeds and with this, I had the challenge of looking for a new playgroup Fraser could attend. I researched the good ones, and we settled for a little one close by to where we lived. Fraser was given the choice to do four mornings but I opted for just a couple of mornings. I felt that he was happier at home and the choice of being able to keep him at home with me before school started in September was appealing. The months whisked by in a blur. Before we knew it, we were preparing him for primary school.

Fraser was a summer baby and was, therefore, due to start in reception class aged just four. I didn't feel like he was really ready to start school, he seemed so young but at the same time Fraser was excited about starting "big boy school". I still to this day wish I could have just kept him at home with me. Little did we know what was just around the corner that would impact our lives in a way we couldn't have foreseen.

Chapter 2 – Starting School

We prepared Fraser for his new school transition. We had bought his new uniform, new bag and spoke about how school would feel. Fraser was very excited and not nervous at all. He was very focused on what was going to happen and seemed eager to start. Other parents would ask me if we had spoken a lot with Fraser about preparing him for school, but his confidence shone so I figured there would be no need to keep going on about his new transition and would let nature take its course and go with the flow!

I remember his first day at school clearly. Nigel had taken the morning off work so that he could come with Fraser and me. I took a photo that morning after we had stepped out of the car and started on the walk up to the school gates. It shows Fraser holding Nigel's hand, taken from behind with Fraser clutching his school book bag in the other hand. For most parents, this picture would represent a milestone happy memory. A photo they could look at with fondness and compare it with how far their child had come since then; the successes and achievements. When I look at it, it holds an air of sadness for me. It was a severe transition for Fraser into a world of rigid discipline that his brain simply couldn't adjust to. So whilst the first day itself was a happy time it was also the start of a journey we could never have predicted.

We walked through the school gates that morning, Dad holding Fraser's hand into the playground that had yet to be packed with kids from the other years. As we walked across the grey tarmac, Fraser seemed too small to be in this big environment. Fraser's classroom was at the far side of the school, at the very edge of the playground where it stopped and gave way to a lush green sports field. As we approached the classroom door we were greeted by a smiling lady who introduced herself as the reception class teacher. On this first day, we would be allowed to stay with Fraser until he had settled. Once he was in the classroom Fraser made a beeline for the building bricks and we sat with him for a short while as he delved into making some sort of construction. He seemed relaxed enough and glancing at Nigel, I tilted my head towards the door indicating that maybe this was the best time for us to leave.

I told Fraser that mummy and daddy would go now and he answered with a simple but assured "ok". We both kissed him on the head and strode back towards the classroom door, making our way past the other children that had started to fill the classroom. On the way back to the car, Nigel and I remarked how grown up he had seemed to let us go like that and we hoped this was a new confidence in him that would flourish throughout his school years.

Later that day, I nervously approached the school to collect him, hoping that he'd enjoyed his first day and hadn't got upset at any point. My mind was immediately put to rest when I popped my head around the classroom door. The teacher grinned at me and said how they would have no problems with

Fraser. He was a delight and had been a star pupil all day. The first week or so continued like this and I was so relieved. He was settling in well and as parents, we were so happy that he seemed to be taking school in his stride.

Towards the end of the second week at school, I walked through the playground as usual on my way to collect Fraser. Standing outside the classroom, I was excited as I waited for my little boy to run out, so he could share with me all the things that he had done that day. This time though, things went a little bit differently. The classroom door opened as usual and the teacher began her usual routine of searching out the parents so that one by one, she could let each child leave the classroom and go home. Gradually each child trickled out and wandered off with their parents into the mild autumn afternoon. It wasn't long before I glanced around me and noticed that I was the only parent left stood there. The teacher popped her head out of the door again and raising her eyebrows, gestured for me to come over to her, "Mrs Stott – can I have a word?", she said. I walked over to where the teacher, and now Fraser stood in the classroom doorway. The teacher had lost her pleasant tone and looked at me sternly.

"Mrs Stott … this afternoon, Fraser would not come out of the construction area when he was asked to move on to the next activity. He refused to play in the kitchen area. Your child became so angry we had to remove him from the class. Can you explain to Fraser that he must learn to play with others on different activities and he can't have it all his own way!"

I looked down at Fraser who looked back at me with sorrowful eyes. I still thought he was very young, and it seemed to me at the time, that this young boy didn't really understand that he needed to share and listen to instructions. I apologised to his teacher and agreed that I would speak to him at home. Fraser and I walked back to the car and I have to admit I felt a little sorry for the small boy walking beside me. He was still just four years old and thrown into a classroom environment with some children nearly a year older than him. Once we reached home, I had a brief conversation with him about what had happened at school. He seemed reluctant to talk about it in any detail and I wasn't going to make him. This little boy had been through enough for one day and he didn't need me reminding him of it all again. I spoke to Nigel when he came home from work and we both agreed it must be an age thing. We would speak to him if things continued but for now, we just thought it was a one-off and there was no point in making a big thing out of it. After all, I didn't want to see a downward spiral when he was so eager to start his new transition.

It didn't end there, however. As the days rolled on, I began getting called over by the teacher at the end of school more often. It started out happening once a week, sometimes more. The incidents at this stage were never more than insubordination and resistance to instructions. To be truthful, I wasn't particularly concerned, and I didn't think it was anything different to how other kids would behave at times. The teacher was adamant that his behaviour was not appropriate. We had placed Fraser in a

Catholic school that had an outstanding Ofsted report. Places were highly contended, and we counted ourselves lucky to have secured him a place there. There did seem, however, to be a large emphasis on conformity and the routine was rigid.

The day would start with a morning prayer, Fraser made the sign of the cross with his arms slightly different to others – which was brought to our attention. It seemed trivial to us but not the school. The teacher explained that this wasn't the only misdemeanour that wasn't acceptable. It was explained to us that when the class finished prayer they went to sit on the carpet. During this time, however, Fraser would be looking elsewhere and fidgeting. The teacher explained to us that she had told Fraser to pay attention numerous times but he simply paid her no regard. Unknown to anyone at this stage, Fraser would be experiencing extreme anxiety during these times and had little control of how his body and senses reacted. Fraser was and is very intelligent, but because he wasn't giving the teacher eye contact this would be taken as a sign that he wasn't paying attention. In one incident, the teacher told us how she had scolded Fraser for not looking her in the eye when she was speaking to him. He had been forced to make eye contact with the teacher which is so hard for many with autism to do, let alone an autistic child of just four years old. Of course, nobody knew this yet. Instead, our son was fast developing a label of the "naughty boy".

As time went on, the school also pointed out how they believed Fraser was being awkward at lunchtimes. "Fraser seems to take such a long time eating his lunch and he is missing time playing with the other children. If he carries on like this he is not going to make any friends". We are liberal parents and believe that our child should have their own personality. To this day we are so proud of Fraser's uniqueness but his strong personality and his desire to do things his way didn't go down well at school. I guess as soon as he walked through the school gates each morning this was working against him.

The complaints from school were regular and happened most days. As time went on, I began to feel exhausted, I couldn't understand why my child wasn't settling. We were starting to become desperate for answers and at one point, I thought we had discovered the reason behind it all.

We noticed how Fraser seemed to have a constant cold. We would frequently visit our GP and more often than not, leave clutching a prescription for a course of antibiotics. At this point, Fraser was going into school three weeks out of four with a blocked-up nose or an ear infection. Initially, we put it down to mixing with other children and the inevitable spread of bugs in school environments. The constant feeling of being unwell was having an impact on Fraser too. He would cry tears of frustration at not being able to breathe through his nose yet again. On top of this, he was putting up with so many demands at school and looked exhausted most of the time. My heart sank sending him there each morning. I would see the parents who had clingy children on the first day walk away from the school gates happy and confident that their child had quickly transitioned into school. My confident bright little boy was going the complete opposite way. I couldn't wait to collect Fraser each day and wrap him in my arms and get him home to somewhere he felt safe and loved.

At this stage, the incidents were still centred around Fraser's refusal to do as he was told. They weren't serious as such, just enough to be disruptive but nothing that required anything more than a reprimand.

One afternoon, I was at home doing the cleaning. It was a murky and cloudy day, the kind of day where you decide to stay at home and clean the house from top to bottom.

Whilst cleaning the bedroom, I could hear my mobile phone ringing out in the dining room. I sighed, annoyed at having my routine interrupted and ran down the stairs to answer the call. I didn't realise that things were about to get much, much worse. The call shocked me. It saddens me now thinking about it.

As my phone came into sight I recognised the school phone number emblazoned across the iPhone display. I slid my finger across the screen and put the phone to my ear, "Hello?", I started …

The female voice at the other end spoke calmly but with concern. "Mrs Stott, we have Fraser in the hallway at school, he has ripped drawings from the displays on the walls, he has also tried to tear his clothes from himself. He is clearly distressed and screaming, we are really not sure what to do, could you come to the school please?"

I said something about being deeply shocked and distressed to hear that my son was in such an emotional state. Was he ok now? What has happened? I was thinking in my head how much my son just needed me there right now. All he needed was for someone to go down onto his level and wrap their arms around him and care for him. I hung up the phone, quickly slid on my shoes and hastily grabbed the car keys.

As I drove over to the school, I pictured the situation my son was in and hoped the staff weren't being stern with him. I couldn't help but wonder why he was acting this way at school as he had never shown this type of behaviour at home, so I could only guess something very distressing had happened. When I arrived at school I half-ran towards the reception door, pressed the buzzer and was quickly let through. The headteacher greeted me in the reception area and took me through to their office where my small, beautiful boy now sat with tear stains under his eyes. He had calmed down but looked sad and a little confused.

The headteacher began explaining what had happened but it wasn't really going in as my head was spinning. All I knew is that I needed to get my boy home. The school couldn't explain what had caused Fraser to behave that way and Fraser couldn't remember much either.

Still thinking that these episodes may be related to a problem with his ears, I knew I needed to push harder at the doctors for answers and get to the bottom of why my child was living on antibiotics half of the month. Maybe he couldn't hear and was in pain constantly at school, how can a child comply when they feel so poorly all the time? In the end, Fraser was seen by an ear, throat and nose specialist. They determined that his adenoids were quite large and advised that it was best to have these removed. He would also need grommets placed in his ears to ensure there was no build-up of fluid. Before long, the hospital appointment date arrived, and we began the process of preparing Fraser for his operation.

The process the NHS goes through to prepare a child for surgery is actually quite good and well thought out. A week or so before his surgery, we took Fraser along to the hospital where a nice lady explained to Fraser exactly what would happen. She showed him the mask he might be asked to wear if the injection didn't make him sleepy enough. We were given a booklet that told the story of a bear who had to go into hospital which Fraser could follow through and read. He was only five years old at this stage but seemed relaxed enough when finally, the day of the operation arrived, and we took him to the hospital.

The date of the operation couldn't have been timed any worse for us. We had been in the process of buying a new house and the day of his operation was the same day the house purchase was due to complete.

However, this came second place as we focused on our little boy that day. I was praying that after the operation things would change. We would have back the boy that we saw at the beginning of the school reception year. I would then be able to return to school with Fraser and show that in fact all along, he couldn't comply with their rules because he couldn't hear properly! I remember collecting Fraser most days in a drained state with residue all over his sleeves and his face filthy where he couldn't wipe his nose properly, his eyes were full, and I was praying that these days would vanish.

So there we were, sat in the hospital and feeling pretty anxious. A number of things were playing out through our minds. How were we going to get Fraser anaesthetised and how would we persuade him that the needle wouldn't hurt (even though he had numbing cream on)? We seemed to sit with Fraser in his bed on the ward for hours, waiting for him to be collected so that he could be taken down to the operating theatre. There had been a delay so we had to wait for an extra hour when finally, the nurses came to take him down. We had already agreed that Nigel would go down with him whilst I stayed on the ward. The plan was to distract Fraser by letting him play some games on an iPad while the general anaesthetic was administered by injection.

Once Nigel and Fraser were out of sight, I sat there on the hospital ward on my own waiting for Nigel to return. After about 25 minutes, Nigel returned looking downtrodden and upset. Nigel explained that things had gone well at first. Fraser seemed almost oblivious to the injection he received but he just didn't fall asleep. The doctor determined that the only thing they could do was to give him gas via a mask instead. A few seconds after the mask was applied, Fraser started to panic and was lashing out trying to remove the mask. Nigel had to go through the terrible experience of holding his son down whilst at the same time trying to calm him before the gas finally took hold. There is nothing worse than the feeling of fighting against your son, him not understanding why the person who loves him so much is doing such a thing. I wouldn't have been able to cope with that situation. Just listening to Nigel telling me what happened made me feel physically sick.

An hour or so later and we were sat in a small waiting room near the operating theatre with the other parents who were also waiting for their children to come out of surgery. My mobile phone started to ring, and I recognised my solicitor's number on the display. She was calling to announce that the purchase of our new house had completed, and we would be moving to a new house tomorrow! At least something was going our way that day.

Each time a child was starting to awaken from their general anaesthetic, the nurse would call for the parents over a speaker in the waiting room. One by one the parents were called and calmly walked out of the room and down the corridor to be with their child. Before long, a voice came over that speaker, asking for the parents of Fraser Stott to come through. However, as soon as the nurse started speaking we could hear Fraser's screams in the background – immediately recognisable. I looked over at Nigel and gasped "It's Fraser!" and with that, we both shot up from our seats and down the hospital corridor. Outside the recovery room doors, we hit the access button and the door was opened by an ashen-faced nurse. We quickly barged past to where the screams were coming from. When we reached Fraser, we were shocked to see him rolling around on a stretcher. His eyes were wide in terror and his face was in shock like he didn't recognise us. We immediately held him to try and calm him down, but he continued screaming and fighting against our attempts. It was like he didn't see us - like we weren't there.

This seemed to go on for ages but in reality, was probably only two minutes. I was starting to get upset because we couldn't settle him, he was strong and trying to fight out of Nigel's arms. I looked at the nurse to question what we should do. I was scared, he wasn't waking up like the other children around him, other children appeared just groggy, but not mine, he was rolling around and didn't seem to know what was going on. The nurse suggested that they may need to put him back to sleep by giving him a sedative to calm him down. Luckily, a doctor rushed into the room, swiftly requesting that all the lights should be dimmed. The minute the lights were turned low was the minute Fraser showed instant relief and calmed down. Luckily, we didn't need to do anymore apart from sit in the dark and rock him like a baby and comfort him. He knew he was now safe and was happy to rest in my arms. I will never forget the look Fraser gave me, it was a sign of relief, he raised his arm and stroked my face, his big brown eyes stared deep into mine. Fraser said things seemed a lot louder, he looked at me and told me he loved me. I had never felt such a loving affectionate moment between us both, I had my little boy back.

Fraser had glue ear and subsequently, a slight loss of hearing before they operated. After the operation, his hearing improved and so did the constant runny noses and earache. I was so happy that we made the decision to have the operation as I firmly believed this was the problem all along. Now this was done, I was looking forward to seeing a happier boy that would get along so much better at school. Fraser was off school for a couple of weeks after the op and we settled into our new house. I was so looking forward to the new school year as we would now see a change in Fraser. With the operation behind him we now had a chance to get him back into school more positive than ever.

Chapter 3 – Year 1 and a Fresh Start

We were advised that year one would be more structured and after seeing how Fraser didn't seem to like the lack of structure in reception, we believed this would suit him too. The first few weeks seemed to go well, Fraser was enjoying a curriculum that was more focused on learning than play. I convinced myself the issues in reception must have been down to one of two things; either reception class at the school was just too strict for a four-year-old or it was due to my son being poorly throughout reception. I was convinced again that the school we had Fraser in was the right setting, the Ofsted report was outstanding, and the parents were a good bunch.

As we started those first tentative weeks in year one everything seemed to be working out. I really believed we had turned a corner. We had a few off days but nothing in comparison to how it was in reception. Fraser was learning, and his health was much better with no snotty noses and being loaded with medicine constantly. Fraser was learning along with the other children and took a keen interest in reading. We were sailing through books each evening and learning to spell for the tests on a Friday. He was receiving good marks in these. I really felt like this was a turning point.

The class teacher told me how things had improved but they were still concerned about how Fraser may progress, there were still some minor issues but if Fraser could address them he could sail through school. It seemed like the teachers were still not sure on how Fraser was going to turn out and they didn't seem as confident as me. It seemed like they were holding back a little. Maybe they didn't want to build my hopes up as they sensed how anxious I was in reception being called into the class most afternoons?

We managed to get through half of year one before I was greeted by his new teacher who was clutching an envelope, she took me to the corner of the playground and was very gentle with me, leading me by the hand. She looked at me with a concerned expression on her face but I could also tell that she wasn't judging me or Fraser. She was a mum herself. I felt like she was talking to me parent to parent rather than as a teacher. I felt that she wasn't judging my parenting and didn't see me as bringing up a spoilt child, she had compassion and from that moment I felt like she didn't think I was to blame, but there on the playground, she had to tell me some news that she said may upset me.

Whilst she held my hand and handed me the envelope, she explained that school had needed to restrain Fraser that day. She explained that it wasn't in a way that hurt him but was only stopping him from hurting others or himself. She explained that the paper would show me where a teacher had to hold Fraser when he had gone into a meltdown, that it was procedure to have it in writing and I would receive a copy if it ever happened again. They only restrained children as a last resort and school did not like to do this. I felt rather sad thinking that an adult was holding my baby boy this way whilst he was in a distressed state. I figured though that it would be a one-off situation.

The teacher asked if we had considered contacting the doctor with regard to some of the day to day issues that were starting to occur. The teacher began telling me that Fraser seemed to be struggling again, she noticed that he looked anxious as soon as he entered the cloakroom in the morning and that he struggled to take his coat off. He seemed to be in a fluster and she told me that she had moved his coat peg to the corner of the cloakroom, so he has a little more space to get his coat off. She said that Fraser was struggling with the crowd of children who were excited to get into class, pushing one another to get to their desk.

She also explained to me that Fraser was reacting negatively if he wasn't allowed to help take the class register in the morning, which was a simple task that each child took it in turn to do. If Fraser wasn't chosen to take the class register, he would begin to throw things – pencils and rubbers in a temper. It seemed that Fraser wanted a purpose each morning. He enjoyed the regular routine of this job, but the teachers told me that it would be unfair for the other pupils if he was chosen to do this each morning. Even queuing in the line at the beginning of school started to become a problem. One push from another child, invading Fraser's space, and he would just explode like a coke bottle that had been shaken up. Most mornings were starting to become a battle. Luckily, we were normally the first on the playground as I dropped my eldest at high school thirty minutes before school started for Fraser, so we got a space at the front of the queue. Fraser would stand and guard his place like a little soldier. The teacher would come to collect the children to march them into class and I would be waiting to give them the thumbs up to signal that the morning so far had been ok. The teacher would always greet Fraser with a smile and a "good morning Fraser". Fraser would look the complete opposite way, avoiding eye contact. Looking back at this now, maybe the school suspected there were underlying issues regarding his behaviour but couldn't say anything outright?

Chapter 4 – Getting a Diagnosis

We booked an appointment with our GP to explain the problems we were having with Fraser. It's an odd situation to be in, as for the first time, I was going to see our GP with a list of behaviours rather than symptoms. At the doctor's surgery, I always feel time pressured but there was so much to tell. Sat there in the waiting room, I was trying to put everything into a coherent and chronological order in my head, whilst glancing at the red LED sign above the reception desk waiting for Fraser's name to appear so that we could go through.

Stepping into the GP's room, I blurted out the whole story from start to finish. The signs at playgroup, his operation and the problems we were having at school. The male GP sat there patiently waiting for me to finish whilst looking at me attentively through his glasses. When I finally stopped to take a breath, he smiled but then explained that due to Fraser being so young it could simply be that he was overwhelmed with his new situation. It was still early days at school and he wasn't used to the routine. With a sympathetic smile he suggested that we should give it a little longer, Fraser would surely become accustomed to the school routine before long. I looked at Fraser sat there beside me and reluctantly accepted the doctor's response. I left the room deflated. I knew there was something else happening but couldn't explain it myself.

By this point, I was becoming more determined to find an answer. Call it instinct but I knew something else was going on in that little boy's head. Around this time, I started talking to one of the other school mums, Zoe. In the playground one day, I was explaining to Zoe the issues that we had with Fraser at school but also some of the traits that I hold dear to this day, such as his quirky sense of humour. Zoe started to tell me how a friend of hers had a son that had recently been diagnosed with autism spectrum disorder (ASD). Zoe recognised some of those traits in Fraser and suggested that I may want to look deeper into this.

Intrigued and with some hope building in me, I went back home and for the next three hours, I researched everything I could on autism. I fed Google with questions related to autism behaviours and read spellbound at the answers. To my amazement, a lot of the behaviours and nuances were exactly those I was seeing in Fraser! That night, I learned that autism was more of a spectrum, with children and adults affected to varying degrees. With a growing sense of intrigue, I read through the characteristics of ASD children.

- preferring to play alone, rather than asking others to play with them;

- not enjoying situations that most children of their age like, such as birthday parties;

- avoiding eye contact;

- having repetitive movements, such as flapping their hands;

- preferring to have a familiar routine and getting very upset if there are changes to this routine;

- seeming to talk "at" people, rather than sharing a two-way conversation.

These described my boy to an absolute tee! That night, I was sure we had found the answer to the problems my boy had to endure, and I was so happy. To me, autism is not something that limited my son. It has given him so many endearing and pragmatic qualities and I would not have him any other way. Nowadays, it's funny how some people react when you tell them that you have an autistic child. A lot of people don't really know much about autism and aren't sure whether to be sympathetic or not. It's like they're frightened to offend you by appearing sympathetic in case it comes across as condescending. Likewise, they're afraid to appear too unsympathetic in case it appears like they don't care.

It's odd because as soon as I read all about ASD and saw the similarities with Fraser, it never entered my mind that it could be anything different. There was no long period of digesting the information and gradual acceptance. I just knew.

I wrote furiously in my notebook all the traits that matched Fraser so that I could take this back to the doctors. Surely, they would have to agree with me and refer him for a formal diagnosis. There was no doubt in my mind that Fraser had autism, I needed to get that message across to everyone else and push for what we believed. I needed this diagnosis so people who were going to be working with Fraser in the future understood him and he was not going to be treated as a naughty boy for the rest of his school life. He would finally be understood.

When Nigel came home that night, I explained to him what I had found. He seemed interested but ambivalent. He agreed that the traits matched Fraser, but Nigel can be much more analytical than me. He isn't always quite so ready to accept the information given to him and needs longer to digest it. We both agreed however that it was something that needed pursuing.

My second trip to the doctor had a completely different dynamic. I decided to approach the school before I went and secured from them a letter to explain how unsettled Fraser was at school and their support for moving ahead with an autism assessment. I was no longer asking for the doctor's opinion. I set out what I believed along with my evidence and asked how we began the process of getting an autism diagnosis. Being quite forthright with the doctor in this respect was important and was key to moving Fraser along to the next stage.

The doctor listened to us and agreed to make a referral to the Child and Adolescent Mental Health Service (CAMHS). CAMHS is a term for the NHS services that includes psychiatrists, psychologists and occupational therapists. They exist to provide all manner of mental health services to young people and do a fantastic job, though they are under a lot of pressure. We were finally on our way to getting

Fraser the help and support he needed but I wasn't prepared for how long all this was going to take.

Shortly after visiting the doctor, we received a call from MindMate. MindMate is specific to Leeds only and in our case, acted as an access gateway or signpost service to other NHS mental health services in the Leeds area. They felt a little bit like the gatekeepers to CAMHS but were very helpful. At various points in our journey, it seems like we've always been directed through MindMate before getting to the service we need. The conversation I had with the pleasant chap from MindMate was brief as they acknowledged that we were going down the correct route for my son, given his situation and that he was now on the waiting list to be seen by CAMHS. We were warned though that the waiting list was extremely long, and it could take around a year to get a diagnosis!

The wait was on, but we were at least on the right path. Things were not improving at school and other parents were starting to complain about Fraser both to the school and directly to me. Fraser was getting into a habit of swearing out loud in school assemblies and at staff. He was becoming increasingly more volatile and lashing out at the children and staff too.

When I heard about the complaints that had been made by the other parents I wished I could explain to them that I was going through diagnosis and Fraser would get the help he deserved soon. The teachers did a great job but I felt that they also needed better support too. At this stage, I did feel like they were also overwhelmed. None of the staff had ever come across a child that behaved this way and the default response was to reprimand. This was never going to work but at the same time, without a diagnosis, it is very difficult to start engaging Fraser in a different way.

The routine of walking onto the playground was a mission itself at this point. I started to feel like the other parents were talking about the behaviours that Fraser was displaying in class and I was starting to feel more paranoid every time I walked through that playground. It was so difficult as I couldn't turn his autism off and couldn't expect him to either. Fraser's autism wasn't like a light switch though I knew his mood swings could be as fast.

I wished I could explain that my son finds it hard to understand feelings and emotions, he may then shout because he is frustrated. Sadly, until we got the help and support in place he would be left with this outcome. We were in the process of going through an assessment that would hopefully lead to a diagnosis and understanding is what we needed, but then it's difficult for others to know the things that you know.

I wondered if the other parents knew how hard it was for me to walk into school knowing that my child wasn't coping? Did they know that I was deeply hurt and upset when my child had upset another a child? Did they know that we were trying our best to get the help Fraser needed and that alone was not easy?

Chapter 5 - Siblings

At this time, things were very tough for my eldest son Tyler. He was 14 back then and witnessed Fraser being treat very differently to how he was brought up. Tyler grew up with a very traditional parenting style - if you're naughty there is a naughty step and if you didn't behave well you would get things taken away from you. However, there weren't any problems with Tyler at school. He was a grounded child and very easy going, we brought Tyler up very well so he knew right from wrong, but Tyler didn't have autism and wasn't facing any of the battles that Fraser had and still faces to this day.

Tyler was still a child himself at this point and trying to explain how different his brother is to him and why we allowed Fraser more leniency, was tricky for him to understand.

I was trying to get my head around autism. I spent countless hours reading bookings and trawling through Facebook groups with questions, but I couldn't expect Tyler to do so. Tyler was interested in boy stuff - playing football, playing with his friends at the local park and he certainly wasn't interested in researching why his brother was acting differently to the way he did.

By this time, Fraser was ruling the roost and had a

streak in him that meant he always wanted to be better than Tyler. If Tyler told Fraser about something he had achieved, Fraser would say he could do it better.

Fraser was taking up more of our time and attention with the behaviours he was displaying, so I guess Tyler felt like he was getting shoved aside a little.

If we decided to watch a family film Fraser had to have the final say on what we watched. If he didn't get his own way Fraser would go into meltdown due to not being in control of the situation. Time after time we had no option but to give in and let him have his own way. Even down to playing a board game as a family, if Tyler won his enjoyment at winning would be immediately taken away by Fraser's triggered meltdown due to not winning. Fraser had a strong desire to win and couldn't accept it when others won.

Tyler's dad lived in York, about 25 miles from Leeds. Tyler would go and visit his dad every other weekend and I believed this was a saviour for Tyler. It was somewhere he could go to get that one to one attention. It was also an opportunity for a little respite from Fraser because home was becoming a tough place with all the challenges we were facing with Fraser's behaviour and the problems at school.

Home wasn't a happy place during this time. It was like walking on eggshells and we were trying to work out how to turn things around - especially during the school week. It started at breakfast time, with me nagging Tyler to get out of bed and get dressed. On the other hand, we allowed Fraser to come down to the kitchen in his pyjamas and then I would dress him whilst he was watching TV. I needed mornings to be as calm as they could be. I knew Fraser couldn't cope with demands. The more I asked him to do something the more anxious he became. Fraser would be in an anxious state at school and I figured we needed to try and make the morning less stressful. As you can imagine, Tyler is rolling his eyes when he comes downstairs to see Fraser sat in the kitchen still in his pyjamas, relaxed, watching his favourite YouTuber. Then, later on, he sees me crouched on the floor tucking Fraser's T-shirt into his trousers. "Why can't Fraser do that himself mum?" I ignore him and carry on getting Fraser dressed. I didn't have the energy to explain the reasons why I was trying to keep the peace this early in the day. I also didn't want Fraser to feel like he wasn't capable and pick up that his brother was questioning him as this would only cause Fraser to explode. Sometimes saying nothing at all was the best way.

I remember one particular day I had gone to pick Fraser up and was told it had been another bad day for him. Upon being told this news for the umpteenth time I could feel my eyes filling with water but I didn't want Fraser to see me get upset. It upset him to see me that way, he would feel guilty when he saw me cry - especially at school. He is a bright boy and knows it must be related to something he has done. I held back my tears after spending the last 20 minutes in the classroom sat on the small stools around a tiny desk, my knees knocking against the desk and my body shaking inside. I didn't feel it was right for Fraser to be sat in the middle of us, but it was too late as the teacher went into full flow detailing the incident that had happened earlier that day. Fraser had thrown a pencil across the room in frustration. The pencil hit a child in class and they had to remove Fraser from the room. Fraser wasn't showing "kind hands" as the school called it. Thinking about it now, Fraser wouldn't have even known in that moment that the pencil was going to hit a child, and throwing an object was him releasing his frustration. Fraser's lagging skills meant he understood his own feelings but found it difficult to understand how others may feel. Once he experiences a teacher removing him from class and giving him orders, he is in fight or flight mode. This time it was fight mode during which he shouted abuse at the teacher, calling her "a big fat dumb idiot".

After speaking with the teacher, we walked back to the car and at this point, I am trying to calm Fraser down. Tyler was already in the car and sensed that Fraser's school day hadn't gone well. There was an atmosphere as we approached and the length of time that it took to collect Fraser from class was a sure sign to Tyler that something wasn't right. Tyler asked Fraser: "What's happened today?" Fraser's face screwed up, his arms crossed. He was still angry and upset at why no one could understand him. I also felt the same way. As I sat there in the driver's seat, I thought that there must be a reason for Fraser's behaviours. As time went on we began to realise that Fraser also had sensory issues around touch – being touched by others sometimes felt almost like an electric shock to him. When he was held or restrained by teachers this was sometimes exasperating the situation. I just wished the teachers had the time to figure it out and help him. Tyler's question only worsened the situation again as I heard Fraser shout at him: "I have been told off again because I called the teacher a stupid dumb idiot because she didn't believe me when I told her that the ball at playtime was kicked at me and it hurt and the other children did it on purpose. Then the dinner lady blew the whistle close to me and it was noisy, then I went back into the classroom and was told to stop crying so I got angry and threw my pencil and it hit Annie Smith on the head! So the teacher then grabbed me and made me sit outside away from class!"

Tyler exhaled deeply and then started to try and tell Fraser how he shouldn't talk to the teacher in that way and really he shouldn't be throwing his pencils. He then looked around at me and asked what I was going to do? I replied: "Nothing, Tyler". Tyler looked at me in shock. He slumped back into his seat and shook his head. "If that was me and I had done that at school today you would have taken something away from me, it's not fair".

I couldn't start to educate Tyler on Fraser's sensitivity to touch, he wouldn't understand. I had told Tyler quite a lot about Fraser's sensory profile, however - he didn't really get it. Tyler didn't understand how Fraser was made to feel very excluded from his peers. Tyler was a different child that grew up with a good group of friends around him, he would have never felt that feeling of isolation – taken by a teacher to work outside on a desk away from his peer group or even in a different room.

Over time I could explain to Tyler more about consequences and the reasons we had to change our parenting style. At school, the majority of the time I knew Fraser wasn't to blame. The school was a mainstream setting and it simply wasn't prepared for an autistic/PDA child, a profile that they would rarely come across. It would be unfair to take things away from Fraser due to his difficulties at school. He would be left with nothing if that was the case.

The difference was that Tyler may have done something wrong once in two months, whilst Fraser had an incident most days. Don't get me wrong, at the beginning we did take things away. Like any other parent, we believed that consequences such as taking the Xbox away, or missing storytime on an evening would change our son's behaviour, but this was different. We didn't understand Fraser enough at that point to realise that this would have the opposite of the desired effect. It would cause his anxiety to rise and result in yet another meltdown.

Every day walking into school, he would start to panic. His hands would start to flap and he would ask me if storytime would be taken away that evening if something bad happened at school. I began to pick Fraser up from school with him begging me not to take anything away, it was soul-destroying. When Fraser was punished at school I came to the conclusion that what happened at school stayed at school. Bringing the problem and guilt back to our once happy home was destroying us all.

As you guessed though, it caused some confusion for Tyler as he was punished for things and then felt like Fraser would and could get away with anything, it wasn't fair. I could tell that Tyler didn't quite understand but I knew in time he would, once I had a diagnosis I could talk with Tyler in the hope that he would understand more the older he grew.

I was hoping once we received a diagnosis someone may be able to help us all as a family.

Particularly to help Tyler understand the reasons why, as parents, we had to change the way we parented to keep Fraser's anxiety at bay. We weren't just treating his little brother differently because he was valued any more than him.

Chapter 6 – In Limbo Land

Life had to carry on and over time we discovered ways to help Fraser cope through our own research, before receiving any professional help. I kept hoping that he was moving up the list for diagnosis and our turn was close.

Fraser was at the age where children would have class parties and that included his own parties too! In fact, I think the only party that actually seemed to go well for him was his own, partly because he was getting all the attention. However, other children's parties were a nightmare.

Fraser's sensory profile stood out like a sore thumb at a birthday party, the noise from the excitement of the children would be too much for him. We would look over and see him sat alone, his hands over his ears trying to block out the noise. Football parties didn't go as planned, with Fraser's sensitivity to touch every time the ball hit him that was it - he would immediately run off in floods of tears. Pass the parcel was the worst. I would see him flapping his arms in excitement as the present got closer to him. Then suddenly, the music would stop before the parcel reached him and a major meltdown quickly ensued. He would shout out loud that it wasn't fair, I would then skip over the other children to lead him to one side of the room to try and explain the rules. I tried to ignore the disapproving glances of the other parents. It always looked as though Fraser was a spoilt kid and just didn't like it if he wasn't getting his own way. In the early days, I honestly thought the same myself. We would go to parties and had no idea that Fraser could possibly be autistic. We took the approach that he would have to understand the rules like everyone else and we did leave one party thinking that he couldn't stay because he was just trying to be in control of everybody and every game. He was just this explosive child and took the enjoyment away for everyone.

Looking back, I guess we were very lucky to be invited to the class parties in the early days of Fraser's mainstream life. I have heard of plenty of autistic children that just never get invites. In a way that would have been much easier for me. I dreaded each party invite that landed in his school bag, knowing what was to come, but Fraser didn't, he was always excited to attend a party and I couldn't take that away from him.

I knew the last party we attended at his mainstream school was going to end up being a disaster for him. When the invite landed for the Nerf gun party I couldn't tell him that he couldn't go. All I could do was pre-warn him what the party was about and what would happen at the party. Again, with Fraser's sensitivity to touch, it was about the worst thing he could attend. A load of shouting kids going berserk with guns firing foam pellets in all directions. It was crazy, yet he was so excited I didn't have the heart to refuse. I sat him down before the party and explained that if he wanted to leave the game and sit out at any time he could do. He agreed to this and sure enough, after 15 minutes of being bombarded by the pellets we had tears. It wasn't getting hit by foam pellets that was the problem so much, he was actually braving those being fired in all directions at him. What really upset him was that no child was following the rules of the game properly. Fraser has a very strong sense of what is right and what is wrong (in his world) and felt strongly about all the rule-breaking. He decided to drag himself away from the game just as the party food was being served. Jugs of orange juice were being passed around and the strong smell of the juice was making him wretch. Then came the time to sing happy birthday. The other boys thought it would be funny to scream instead of sing. Yet again Fraser was at the table with his hands over his ears. It's a hard choice as I knew that he was going struggle but I also knew that he would have struggled more being the only child who wasn't going to the party, it's a tough call to make.

We tried to help Fraser in more ways than one to get him involved in socialising him with other children. We tried group swimming lessons, it worked out ok the first few times but then things got worse. Anyone that invaded Fraser's part of the pool would be subjected to his wrath. When the swimming teachers explained to Fraser what they required of him it just sent his head fuzzy. He wanted to swim but trying to swim with a group of other children just didn't work. If Fraser came last at something or if another child did better then him he would immediately show his resentment. We would hear how "rubbish" swimming was or he would simply refuse to listen to the instructor.

Next we tried karate. Nigel had done karate for years when he was younger and enrolled Fraser at the same club, with the same instructor he had had all those years ago. Karate is very discipline-based and when all the students were stood in line to bow to the instructor, sure enough, Fraser was standing out of the line in his own space, dancing and pulling funny faces at himself in the mirrors that surrounded the room. Looking back, we smile at this unique quirkiness he still shows to this day. It was like he was in his own little bubble. Once they started doing some techniques he started throwing himself on the floor. I am unsure what he was there for, but it certainly wasn't karate. After a few weeks, we decided that karate really wasn't for him. This led us on to street dancing ...

I believed that if he had a passion for dancing at karate then we should give the boys street dancing club a go! Anything to try and help him socialise and to form friendships. Dancing was good, he had an understanding teacher - she loved his quirky attitude and the passion he had to learn. I thought we may possibly have our next Billy Elliot and this was it! Dancing was probably the longest hobby he kept with a group of other boys.

He spent most of the lesson looking in the mirror and pulling funny faces to himself but he was happy. He wasn't too keen when he had to hold hands with the other boys but it was ok. Fraser was part of a nice little group that he started to build friendships with. He even did a dance show and took a dancing exam! Things sadly turned worse when tap dancing lessons started to take place in the same room. We believed that the noise was starting to become a bit overwhelming for Fraser. Fraser was starting to get frustrated and would lash out a few times so I would have to go into class and pull him out. It was sad at the time because none of this was his fault, it was just that the noise levels were too much for his senses to cope with. He was deeply sorry as soon as we left the room and his teary big brown eyes would look at me with confusion. Of course, we wouldn't treat it as a punishment and we would go across the road and choose the biggest cake in the coffee shop to munch on in the car on the journey home. Fraser managed for a while but then a couple of new boys joined the group, one was much younger and didn't take the dancing very seriously. Fraser didn't gel with younger children at the best of times but a child that wasn't doing as he was told and wasting his dance lesson was getting too much. Once Fraser is focused on doing something it's very clear cut. Rules are rules and they must be followed. If you don't follow the rules then all hell is going to break loose. I was finding myself having to sit at the side of the dance class tucked in the corner ready for when Fraser would finally blow, to go and rescue him and take him away from the situation. This was happening too many times, so we mutually decided to leave the dance club and start something new.

Whilst we waited in limbo and carried on doing what we did, I got my head stuck in books and searched the internet for local support groups. I needed to find out as much as I could to help Fraser. To this day some of my closest friends are from Facebook groups that I have now met in person, they're the only people that truly understand.

Nigel and I started to discuss how we would approach Fraser about the diagnosis appointments he would soon be attending. Fraser was a bright lad so we knew we had to explain why he was attending the appointments but at the same time it was quite a complicated thing for a young boy to understand. The only thing I could think was to tell him that the school needed to understand better how his brain worked. We could explain to him that is why things weren't going too well at school sometimes and the teachers needed to understand him better. They have never had a child in their school with such a clever brain, and the doctors haven't either, so we need to go to these appointments just to explain how things work so they can put them in their reports. I would always throw a positive about how amazing he was and still is! Fraser seemed happy about this, he seemed happy that the school were going to learn about how his brain worked and how they could understand him a little better!

Time ticked by and then one morning, about eight months after we had first joined the autism diagnosis waiting list the post plopped onto the doormat. I gathered the post together and tore open a rather plain-looking brown envelope. When I saw the CAMHS logo at the top of the page I knew immediately that this was the news we had been waiting for! I quickly scanned the letter and sure enough, the time had come for Fraser to start going through the assessment process. The letter provided a date for our first appointment with CAMHS. It explained there would be two initial appointments and then a final assessment where they would draw their conclusions!

Firstly, we had an appointment with Fraser, myself and Nigel. We were seen by a nice lady who explained the process we would be going through. It was fairly brief and Fraser spent the majority of the time sitting on the chair explaining how school wasn't very good but what he liked to do was play Minecraft and explained his fascination with computers. All the time he spoke, he avoided looking at the lady who had been assigned to us and was asking the questions. If Fraser was uncomfortable and didn't feel relaxed, he would answer the questions by looking at me, expecting me to join in the conversation and then finish the question off. The first appointment went ok. For the first time, we had someone who listened to us and listening was a huge step, it felt like we had finally got someone that was hearing our views and we were going in the right direction.

The second appointment was for just us as parents to attend. In the meantime, the school had completed a few reports so CAMHS had some additional information about Fraser to work from. During that appointment, we met with a nice chap called Ted. He introduced himself as a child psychologist and asked us a lot of detailed questions. After a long discussion about Fraser's behaviours, he asked if we wanted to go ahead with an autism assessment? Of course, we replied! Another waiting list but at least something was going to happen. Even if these were baby steps, we were finally moving forward.

The final step involved a detailed assessment of Fraser. On the day of the assessment, we were nervously sat in the waiting room - myself, Nigel and Fraser. It was a little box room at an NHS clinic not far from our home. It reminded me of a dark dungeon to be honest. It was dull and had a sad feeling to it, but what brightened the room that day was another little boy waiting for his assessment too. He seemed to be with his father and was telling him all about Minecraft and the way he was building his Lego. As if like magic Fraser started to engage with him. The two boys hit it off straight away and we hadn't seen Fraser chatting to another child like this in a long time. When he tried engaging with any peers at school they seemed to get bored of Fraser's conversations after a few minutes, but these two boys were chatting away and laughing together like they had known each other for years and were enjoying every second. Before long, a lady with dark curly hair entered the room followed by Ted, the child psychologist we had met previously. The lady called out the boy's name and off they went into one of the rooms. I leant over to Nigel and whispered: "If that boy doesn't get an autism diagnosis, Fraser is completely not on the spectrum either!" They were like twins.

Before long, the lady with the dark curly hair reappeared and told Fraser it was his turn to go in. I asked how long they would need Fraser for and they told me that it would be around an hour, they would be doing some simple tasks to see how Fraser responded and then we would be told via letter in the following weeks the outcome of their assessment.

So off he went, our little boy with his light brown hair with two complete strangers he had never met before. I wasn't sure how he would cope for an hour, but I told him that mummy and daddy would just be outside the door if he needed us.

Eagerly we waited, though time seemed to go so slow sat in that small, dark waiting room watching the clock tick by. Suddenly after 30 minutes, a flushed cheeked little Fraser appeared at the door. He trots up to me and says he needs to go to the toilet, so I take him there and he tells me that his tummy is hurting and he feels a bit sick. I am guessing it's the anxiety, so I tell the lady and man who are assessing him how he is feeling. They tell me that I can go in the room with him this time as they are nearly finished and even if Fraser couldn't finish they think they have enough now anyway. I opt to go into the room and I take a seat beside him while they play a game. This game is all about objects and the lady holds up an egg, a spoon and a fork. She tells Fraser that she believes the egg is a person and the spoon and the fork are people too. When the lady asks Fraser to make a story up using the objects he makes the story up with exactly what he sees, referring to the objects just as they are – an egg, a spoon and a fork. He couldn't do make-believe. After the game, the lady called it a day and she told Fraser that she'd had a great time with him.

What really struck me is that just before Fraser left, the lady crouched down in front of him. She looked into his eyes and said: "Fraser, you have an amazing brain and don't let anyone else tell you any different". I had a thought that this was maybe her way of telling us all, unofficially, they believed Fraser was on the autistic spectrum – but we still had to wait for the diagnosis result. They told us that in the weeks to come, they would discuss their findings with a panel of experts and a final decision would be made then.

We walked away from that appointment with a high sense of hope that he was his complete true self that day and they would recognise what we knew and help was on its way for us all.

A few weeks later we were preparing for our family holiday and we still hadn't received a letter from CAMHS to confirm whether Fraser was on the autistic spectrum or not. Each morning I would check the letterbox to see if it had arrived but no joy, I couldn't rest knowing that we were going away and didn't have an answer. We had waited too long and I needed to know – the wait was making me feel sick. I thought maybe I should call and chase it up, I might get an answer over the phone. Who knows - it was worth a shot.

I dialled the number on my mobile, half of me didn't want to know but half of me did, it was a strange feeling that was a mixture of nervousness and excitement.

After a couple of frustrating days, it was Ted who finally called me back. I explained to him the situation – we were shortly due to go on holiday and were desperate to know the outcome of the assessment. Ted began talking in a very calm voice: "Ok, I understand Mrs Stott. Well, I can confirm that in our eyes the assessment was very straight forward and clear cut. We have discussed our findings with the panel of experts and we all agree that Fraser has Asperger syndrome, which is part of the autistic spectrum".

He then went on to explain to me a little more about Asperger syndrome: "People with Asperger syndrome experience the world differently to other people", he explained. "It's something that Fraser will have for life".

He then went on to explain that people with Asperger syndrome generally don't have the learning disabilities that other autistic people may have, but there may still be some difficulties in learning that Fraser would experience. He advised that Fraser would need a lot of help, support and understanding.

"I will send you confirmation in the post", he finished. With that, I thanked him so much for all his help. I was elated that we now had something we could work with and the relief in me was evident.

I wasn't sure whether to cry or feel excited that we finally had an answer. It confirmed to me that I wasn't a bad parent. There were reasons for Fraser's behaviours and finally people including us as parents could understand.

Seeing your child breakdown and be so fragile is the hardest thing, but not being able to help and understand was also hard - but now we could take steps in the right direction. I picked up the phone and told Nigel – he too was very relieved that we now had something, an explanation, that we could work with.

Chapter 7 – Sharing the Diagnosis and Taking Action

It was like winning the lottery - finally having something on paper to show school, to prove to them that my son wasn't just naughty and there was a reason behind his behaviour. Even though we had shared our thoughts with the school about how we suspected he had autism, we still felt that it wouldn't be taken seriously without a formal diagnosis.

The pieces had now fit into place like one of Fraser's favourite jigsaw puzzles!

Fraser's autism meant that he didn't play like the other children. In his early days, he was obsessed with making his "inventions" as we called them. Sometimes, he made a line of all his favourite cars or would just play with random objects like my car keys, the phone, a charger, wires – anything! As long as they all linked together like a circuit he was the happiest kid alive! The same with blocks and puzzles. If you stuck him with a group of kids for imaginary play he wouldn't understand it. His brain wasn't wired to pretend that his schoolmates were a nurse or a chef .. the play kitchen wasn't real - it was plastic, why would others play this way? This was the reason for the meltdowns in reception, he was forced to move from something he understood (like a construction set) to play with something that he really didn't understand, so why wouldn't he be upset? He didn't have anyone guiding him or explain to him this thing we call "make-believe". Everything was black and white with Fraser. When a school friend passed him an empty cup to pretend to drink tea he couldn't comprehend it – it wasn't real. Fraser would argue that it wasn't real and look confused. This caused meltdowns, which would inevitably lead to him being whisked from the classroom and into the headteacher's office.

Everything made sense for us now, the extreme reactions to the mundane aspects of school life that most of us take for granted and never struggle with. The part of his brain that would not let him look the teacher in the eye, sit still on the carpet or accept a world of make-believe was the reason he was starting to spend more time outside of the classroom than in it.

One morning we walked down the dreaded path into the school playground. Fraser was holding my hand when I saw one of the older boys looking over at us and whisper to his friend as we wandered by. Intrigued, I asked him what he was whispering about? He seemed happy to tell me that "Fraser is never bothered when he goes to the headteacher's office - it seems to be the place where Fraser hangs out the most". It saddened me, but then I was relieved that it really didn't seem to bother Fraser too much. I think it bothered me more.

I knew we needed to make some significant changes at school, so I requested a meeting with the headteacher, who also happened to be the special educational needs co-ordinator (SENCO) to discuss the adjustments that we could put in place for our son now that we had a diagnosis. I started making out a list of the areas where Fraser struggles and considering his sensory profile, adjustments that we should consider making in the school environment.

The crowded cloakroom was too much for Fraser to handle, he was becoming overwhelmed with the amount of noise and children in such a small and confined space. I wrote down a suggestion that Fraser should be able to have a place at the front of the cloakroom, where there was more space and he could go straight into class without having to fight through the other children. The queue to go into class in a morning was also a problem area. Maybe if he was at the front or the back of the queue he wouldn't feel like his personal space was being invaded and would walk into the school in a more settled manner. Fraser also liked to feel that he had a purpose and was contributing so maybe giving him a job to do, such as taking the class register more frequently would make him focus on his task and make him feel worthy.

So off I went with my list of suggestions on how things could change and how I believed things would become more settled at school. I emailed the SENCO with my ideas.

I had to be fairly clear in my email to the school, we understood Fraser's needs so these weren't so much requests we were making but key requirements. We were not convinced that there was enough appreciation of autism and its complexities within the school and felt compelled to take the lead in ensuring his needs were addressed. A diagnosis of Asperger syndrome only gave us a label, it didn't come bundled with any kind of support or assistance. There were courses on autism available but the waiting lists were around two years long. During this time, I was able to educate myself and became very knowledgeable about autism.

It was around this time we received the news that the headteacher was leaving his role and a new lady would be coming in to replace him and take on the headteacher and SENCO roles. She would be starting in September and would be getting in touch with all parents who had children at the school with special educational needs to introduce herself. This was around the time that Fraser was coming towards the end of year two.

Year two had actually been much calmer for Fraser. He was lucky to have two very good teachers, one of whom was particularly good with Fraser and would always provide him with the additional attention and support he required. Fraser had a very good relationship with them, and we thought that he had finally settled. However, we were unprepared for his transition to year three and the problems that were yet to come.

Chapter 8 - The Guilt

When we received the diagnosis it left a huge pile of guilt on my shoulders. How didn't we guess?

We were blind not to see our son's unique sensory profile from a young age, and how we didn't guess that he was autistic back then I don't know? Then again, we didn't even know there was anything wrong until we started to question things at age six. Perhaps I should rephrase the "anything wrong". It wasn't "wrong" – it was simply his own sensory profile that was different from most children of the same age.

My first child was a laid-back baby who hardly cried, enjoyed being in my arms and was generally very chilled. Fraser, on the other hand, seemed so different, very upset and hard to settle. He would arch his back when I tried to cradle him in my arms so I searched for answers thinking that he may be allergic to the milk formula or maybe it was colic. I know two babies can certainly have different characteristics but even from being inside my tummy I knew this baby was going to be different. I could sense his personality from deep inside me the way he moved and wriggled nonstop – he was going to be a fighter. I felt there was a certain determination and a strong character in there. Little did we know then that we created a unique child that was different in his own ways and whom I would be so proud of in years to come.

We lived in a townhouse from when Fraser was a baby until he was about three years old and I remember clearly how distressed he would become when the neighbour used his lawnmower. Now me being oblivious to the world of autism back then, I would smile over the fence to my neighbour and tell him its fine, my child will get used to it –it's only the lawnmower! Little did I know, my neighbour had a son who also had Asperger syndrome. I guess he might have suspected something before we did. This all happened around the age of two years old. Thinking back, our neighbours were probably trying to drop hints as their understanding was so much clearer than mine, I just thought we had a sensitive child. I feel ever so guilty that I didn't realise what was actually going on.

We picked our first holiday abroad when Fraser was aged four. We chose a hotel that was right on the beach as we thought the children would love this. That was until we left the hotel to go on the sand. As soon as Fraser's feet touched the sand he began crying and screaming, desperate to get the sand off his feet. As completely oblivious parents we looked on, slightly amused and also confused. I argued with Nigel "He's got to get used to it, let him feel the sand, he will be fine". How naive was I!? During the whole holiday we spent days trying to tackle the beach but came to the conclusion that our child just didn't like sand! Again, we were so oblivious to our child's sensory needs. How couldn't we have spotted this yet? *The sensory feeling of sand on his feet, or even hands.*

The holiday souvenir shop did very well from us that week as we had to keep finding new toys for him to play in the sand with. We were hoping that he would get used to it and want to play. Holidays were important to us and still are, Nigel holds down a demanding job and, in my head, I thought it was so important Fraser got used to the sand. For me, the beach and sun make the perfect holiday. Little did we know, and now looking back I think to myself I was a bad mum for not understanding my child.

There were other signs we missed too. Who doesn't like coffee? Well, I'm unsure what I would do without my coffee in a morning. This one makes me cringe thinking about it because *STILL,* the penny hadn't dropped at this point. When Fraser was about five the morning routine consisted of grabbing a coffee en-route to school. As soon as the cups of coffee were in the car, we would hear a gagging noise coming from the back. Looking around, I saw that Fraser's eyes were streaming and he seemed to be completely overwhelmed with the smell. We would explain over and over again that it's only a drink. The smell to us wasn't strong but to him, the smell of coffee was like a rotten egg. We had to stop drinking coffee in the car, his senses were that strong he would be the first to tell us if someone had been in the car with a cup! Again, we had no idea, we just thought our boy was a unique quirky little chap and made adjustments without even knowing a diagnosis was down the path in years to come.

We've been lucky to manage to get out and about as a family and we still do regularly despite his challenges. I am hoping this may long continue though, thank goodness for electronic devices! One of the things we do as a family is to go out to restaurants when we can and although we're much stricter with our diet nowadays, we do like a good Indian! We had heard good reports about a local Indian restaurant and all piled in the car one evening to try it out. We entered the plush marble laden reception area and were quickly shown to our table in the busy restaurant amongst the other guests. No sooner had Fraser sat down he suddenly looked up from the game he'd had his nose stuck into and told us he felt sick. He started making loud gagging noises and looking like he was actually going to be vomit. With that, Nigel quickly rushed him off to the toilet. The first time this happened we left in a rush but once we got home Fraser said he felt fine and had no further problems for the rest of the evening. We ended up with a take away that night but were left wondering whether he could have caught a bug? Keen to go back to the restaurant, we tried a second time a few weeks later. Again, as soon as we were seated the same scenario happened. This time Fraser declared loudly: "This place makes me feel sick!". We rushed through our starters and embarrassingly left the restaurant as others stared at us thinking we had forced a sick child to come out with us!

We gave it one more go. We spoke with our child, pre-warning him that we were going to eat out again, reassuring him that he was fine now and didn't need to act like he was poorly when we got to the restaurant. Third time lucky right? Not at all - we lasted 10 minutes and left. The smell to him was so strong his senses just couldn't tolerate the spicy aroma.

I thought back to the awful school journeys that

we had coming home before he was diagnosed, the teacher called me in daily and I was becoming exhausted. Why was school such an issue, but at home we had a fraction of the issues? We had strops like any child but nothing like the amount the staff were facing at school. I was becoming exhausted collecting Fraser, and the teachers telling me how uncontrollable my son was.

At home, we tried sticker charts and we also tried rewards if Fraser had been good at school all week. It was becoming expensive but worth it if it kept the teachers off my back and Fraser's, however, nothing seemed to work. The incidents continued.

I was exhausted seeing the teacher after school every day, I was exhausted walking back to the car with Fraser in floods of tears telling me how sorry he was and the upset in his eyes, while I myself had water filling up in my eyes, trying my hardest not to fall to pieces before I got to the car. As soon as we were in the car, my tears would just flow. I can hear Fraser now crying in the back seat, explaining how sorry he was. I was confused at the time and all I could ask him was why? Why Fraser are you acting this way to your teachers and your class friends? Please, Fraser, mummy is tired and needs you to start acting a good boy. Fraser would repeat over and over again "I'm sorry, I'm sorry, I'm sorry" ... he didn't like to see me upset but was also confused as to why he was getting so angry and frustrated. I would tell him: "Ok Fraser I know you are sorry, let's leave it there". He still thought I was angry though; my tone was not a happy tone and now from professional reports I know that Fraser struggles to understand the tone of voice. Hindsight is a wonderful thing and I only wished I had known this earlier. Fraser would apologise for the whole of the journey. My head was pounding and I just wanted to reach for a large glass of wine and forget about the day, and the journey home. However, when I got home I couldn't stop thinking of what my poor boy must have been going through, not being understood - even by me. All I knew was that I needed to get us all some help for things to improve.

On these days, once home, Fraser wouldn't calm down and was still upset and frustrated. He had many "bad days" like this. Upon returning home his anxiety was still high and we all needed some space. I remember walking up into my bedroom and sitting behind the door, sobbing hard. I didn't want Fraser to see how upset I was, he didn't seem to understand why he was acting this way at school and neither did I. This was the worst bit. I wish I had known back then what I know now. I could have helped him but I guess every parent isn't provided with a handbook that shows them how to manage a child with ASD?

We needed something to change as I couldn't face year three with all this upset. I could envisage it all already, I would be called over last by the teacher whilst Fraser peered out the window with a sad face and a thumbs down which meant that he'd had a bad day. It was like our own sign language that we built up together. By this point, Fraser had developed a habit of lashing out at the other children when his anxiety was particularly high. After school, the teacher would tend to go over to the parent of the child that Fraser had lashed out at first and explain that there had been an incident between their child and mine. The first few times this happened, I would talk to the parent and apologise in the playground the next day. However, it became such a regular thing that I stopped saying sorry to the parents, they had heard it once before and there was not much more I could do. I wasn't at school to see and stop him doing these things but the guilt of knowing that my child had hurt another child was horrendous. I felt ashamed to walk into the playground and over time I started to stand alone – distancing myself from the other parents.

Chapter 9 - Year 3 with a Bang

Now we had the diagnosis I had to start putting the guilt behind me. I had to focus all my energy on getting the support we all needed. I figured now that we had the diagnosis, Fraser could be understood by the teachers and his peers a little more, and he would no longer have the naughty boy label.

My first point of call was to arrange a meeting with the new headteacher who was also the SENCO. Upon meeting the headteacher for the first time, I was pleasantly surprised by her upbeat and friendly manner. I stepped inside her office and we discussed Fraser's situation. I was shown a piece of paper that contained the details of Fraser's IEP (Individual Educational Plan). An IEP is a document that is designed for children with special educational needs to succeed in their education. An IEP builds on the school curriculum that a child with learning difficulties or disabilities is following and details the strategies being used to meet that child's specific needs. The IEP also had targets for Fraser to aim for. I looked through the targets and wasn't sure what to make of them. They didn't really seem to be focused on his education but at the same time, he was having real difficulty with basic tasks such as writing and maths.

The IEP targets were:

- To have kind hands for 80% of the time (kind hands was the school code for not hitting children or staff);

- To not shout out 60% of the time;

- To be kind to other children in the class;

- To be able to complete maths and English work during the morning.

I was new to all this but I presumed that school had dealt with children on the spectrum before. I believed that whatever way they were going to deal with Fraser, they had done it before and it was going to work. I trusted that they knew what they were doing and for the first time felt included. The school wanted to work with me and I felt like they were wanting to work with us to improve things. In the meeting, we also discussed making adjustments for Fraser to help him cope with the school day better.

- Fraser would be allowed to go into the classroom five minutes before the rest of the class would enter the room;

- Fraser would be given a desk of his own in the classroom so he had space and wasn't frustrated with the children next to him that he may perceive as being too noisy;

- Fraser was also given a desk just outside the classroom in the corridor for when he was finding the classroom too overwhelming;

- He would have access to a sensory box to play with which included a stress ball and other sensory toys;

- Fraser would not be forced to go into assemblies or church as he found that the noise and the environment would raise his stress levels.

I walked away with the little pre-made IEP booklet feeling like we had made progress. At the time all these changes seemed positive and the school were trying to do everything they could to help. What we realised over the next few weeks, however, is that these measures were ostracising Fraser further from his classmates. It was completely unintentional, but it was evident to the rest of his peers that Fraser wasn't really part of their class anymore.

In less than two weeks things still declined even with all these strategies in place.

As parents, we realised that all we were doing was dealing with the symptoms of his behaviour. Fraser's frustration and anxiety was growing fast and the staff had to start restraining him in school. This would be for a variety of reasons - with him attempting to hit staff or pupils or damaging school property. Fraser would be removed from the classroom, in front of all the children and be whisked to the headteacher's office. The war would carry on there - books would go flying, as would the chairs and tables, he was only six years old by this point but had a lot of energy and strength.

Through our own research, we learned how a highly anxious child would drop into fight or flight mode during these times. As humans, our brains are programmed to have one of two responses when it senses extreme danger. In the days of stone age man, this programming helped ensure our survival when we came across a woolly mammoth or sabre tooth tiger. Our brains would sense the danger and determine whether we should run for our lives or stay and fight if there was no escape. A third alternative would have been to freeze, and do nothing. In these modern times, our genetics haven't really changed from thousands of years ago, but the environment has. Fraser's autistic brain mistook his extreme anxiety, due to a lack of understanding about the world, as danger. He couldn't escape the school environment but he sure as hell could put up a fight.

Fraser told me that it only ever made him feel angrier when they used to hold him or escort him to another room. The school were keen to ensure the safety of him and others which we understood but it still didn't stop the upset of knowing that our young boy of six was being physically restrained by adults. The restraining became a regular part of school life and it was very upsetting for us.

We were starting to get confused again around his behaviour. We had his Asperger syndrome diagnosis and had put plans in place to try and address the behaviours that resulted from this. Fraser had the adjustments in class, an IEP, even behaviour sheets with red and green faces that indicated his targets. If he achieved a majority of green faces during the day, he would be rewarded. None of this seemed to be working. In fact, his behaviour was getting more extreme and much, much worse.

He was feeling very singled out at this point, his self-esteem had hit a massive low and as soon as he entered the school gates you could see a mask come on, it was a fighting mask ready for an explosion.

I remember walking through the school gates and into the playground, I gripped Fraser's hand tight. Maybe I imagined it but I felt like everyone was looking at us. Unfortunately, Fraser was getting a reputation within the school and it sometimes felt like all eyes were on us. We would make our way to the classroom door and there we stood, with me wishing that someone would let him in a little bit earlier. That way, Fraser wouldn't look like he was on his own.

We would stand there and wait. In his IEP, the school had agreed that the teacher would come out five minutes before the school bell rang to take Fraser into class early. Five minutes didn't give Fraser much time to get his bag put away, coat off and get seated at his lonely desk. I was hoping that we would have been allowed a little longer to make sure he was settled, I even offered to help to bring him in but I felt that was frowned upon. To add to the mix, on some mornings the teacher would be late which meant that Fraser didn't get the opportunity to get settled before everyone came in. Those days would start with Fraser in high anxiety mode trying to manage the noise around him as the other children rushed into class.

As part of this routine, we would always stand away from the other children and parents whilst we waited for the teacher to let us in and it was at this point that the isolation really hit home. Although, thinking about it, I guess I had a sense of relief that I no longer had to try and make small talk with the other mums. It was hard when the last conversations I had were apologising for Fraser's behaviours towards their children.

We rocked up to our little space and played hopscotch and made games up between ourselves before the teacher let Fraser in.

It was suggested that the charts of the red and green faces may help indicate when incidents were occurring. It seemed that a lot of the red faces were developing over lunchtime. At the time I was very suggestible and went along with most things I was being advised. I treated them as the best approaches that were being put in place by the professionals. It was suggested that Fraser attend the computer club during lunch and seeing as though he had a keen interest, this made sense. The noise in the dining hall was triggering meltdowns which were leading to him being restrained and marched out of the dining hall. The aroma of the food being eaten by the other children had an impact on Fraser. He couldn't stand the smell of juice and the sight of yoghurt (which was all about an aversion to the texture). Sadly, this became a tease, children knew this and would make a big song and dance about what they were eating, especially if they were opening their yoghurt. With Fraser reacting negatively to this and being quite loud, the stern looks from the lunchtime staff would tip Fraser over the edge, to the point where he would then have a meltdown and when this occurred teachers were sent in to drag him out. These are things we didn't know until months later, when we had managed to obtain school records relating to his behaviour under new data protection laws.

I was out one morning after taking Fraser to school. It was 10:50 am and I looked down at my phone. The lively dance music that acts as my ringtone masked the inevitable dread I felt when I saw the school phone number emblazoned on the caller ID. My heart sank as I knew when the school called, it was never good news. I slid the answer call button and the headteacher told me that the school are really struggling with Fraser. They have dealt with autistic children before but have never had anyone like Fraser. She then told me that every child is different, and they understand that, but they just don't know how to cope with him any longer. They had made the decision to exclude Fraser from school for two days as he hit a teacher whilst in a meltdown. I was told it was seemingly over nothing and there was no trigger. I had to come into school right them to collect him, there were also some forms they needed me to sign and they also needed to give me some homework for the next few days.

I remember driving up to the school shaking. When they called me, I was just leaving the woods after taking the dog for a walk and was caked in mud, in my scruffy clothes and wellies. I had quickly dropped the dog off at home and called Nigel to tell him what had happened. Nigel was as shocked as me and asked me to call him back at work once I knew more.

I felt sick, would I be met by my son in meltdown mode, in floods of tears or even possibly being held by teachers in the office? I pulled my car right up to the playground, disregarding the rules on parking. I figured if Fraser was in meltdown I may need to carry him into the car to get him out of that place. When I got there, to my astonishment, my little boy was just sat on a chair in the office with the executive headteacher (who ran two schools in the area). The executive head looked saddened and asked if I was ok? He mentioned that they had never had to do this before, but Fraser's anger had reached an extreme and unacceptable level and they could no longer allow him to hit teachers. As he explained this to me, he could see the upset in my eyes, he offered me a tissue but I declined. I knew I had to keep it together because if I let one tear out that would be the trigger to release all of the tears and that would have just upset Fraser. It was unfair for him to see me that way. Fraser wasn't aware of what was going on, he just thought it was a regular visit to the head's office, where he would throw anything he could see and then they would hold him till he got even angrier and then eventually gave in.

He looked at me in surprise: "Mummy what are you doing here?" I smiled at him softly to show that I wasn't mad but maybe just a little upset and explained that I had come to take him home. School hadn't told him this bit I guessed. They didn't know how to explain it to someone so young, so I had the unique job of trying to explain the reasons why he had to come home with me. I explained that school have told me that you hit a teacher, and the school can't allow you to keep doing this. Fraser then looked at me sadly and confused as if there was a reason for his actions, but his little head couldn't tell me. I explained it was all ok and we just needed to leave.

We got escorted out of the building to the car. As we approached the car, Fraser burst into tears. He said he will miss his Minecraft afterschool club. He started to realise and panicked about what he would miss. I reassured him that it was going to be ok.

As we drove out of the school gates Fraser looked at me and repeatedly told me how sorry he was. I pulled the car over and climbed into the back seat and threw my arms around him. I told him that it wasn't his fault and they don't understand him but I do, his family does … everything was going to be ok. Your mummy will make things better. Everything will be better.

Fraser wasn't accessing much of the curriculum before his exclusion and had refused to write. He was spending 90% of his time outside the classroom, at his special desk, with his stress toys. I was amazed how at home, he suddenly wanted to engage and was willing to learn. On the day of his exclusion, the Executive Head gave me eight sheets of homework to attempt with Fraser whilst he was off. We nailed this in one day with no frustration or anger. We spent the next day having lots of cuddles and having fun. I wasn't going to make his two days at home with me feel like a punishment. I needed to prove that the setting wasn't right for him and this had to change.

The school suggested that on our return, his school peers should understand that he has autism. This would help his classmates understand him better and maybe help them comprehend why Fraser was behaving the way he was.

At this point we hadn't explained to Fraser that he had autism, we had only told Fraser that he had a special brain, a clever brain but that meant he sometimes had trouble understanding things the way everyone else does. With the school keen to communicate Fraser's diagnosis to the class, we were under pressure to explain to Fraser his diagnosis and talk about autism. It was unfair to tell everyone else and for him to find out last. I was quite saddened how quickly we were forced to explain this to Fraser but I kind of understood why the school needed to explain autism to the rest of the children. They needed to know why one of their class friends couldn't always be just like them.

I wanted to tell Fraser all the positives of being autistic. I would never tell him the daily struggles of an autistic person, he knew the struggles – he was facing them every day. I needed to focus on all the positives and explain that autism is not a disease - put simply, his brain was wired differently to others. But oh! This meant he was a unique amazing little boy and his brain was inquisitive, insightful and looked at the world in such a different way compared to mummy's boring brain! We went through all the famous people that had autism and demonstrated how this was a positive thing. We threw every positive thing that we could find at it … we still do now. This wasn't just us trying to make our child feel better. We are so proud of our son who understands aspects of the world in a way we never did at his age.

The school suggested that the class should watch a video about autism to help them appreciate Fraser's challenges. I explained this to Fraser and asked him if he was ok with this. He watched it and said he found the video a bit weird but it was ok, he got some things and thought some were like him. He agreed it was fine to show the class and it may help them understand him.

School said that they would show the class the

video when Fraser was in Lego therapy. This would give the class an opportunity to ask any questions they may have. At the time I still felt it was too soon to be telling the class, seen as though Fraser had just found out, but if Fraser agreed then I was happy to allow this. I personally felt like we had not much choice, school were working hard to accommodate Fraser and no doubt the questions of concerned parents.

I was told that the class took it very well. After the video, the teacher asked each child to mention a good thing about Fraser. Each one did and I actually felt like the children in his class understood, after all, they had lived and grown up with Fraser for three years and to them, nothing had changed.

Chapter 10 - Back to School

After his exclusion, we had walked back into school and Fraser was keen to show the teacher all the work he had done with me whilst he was off. Upon seeing his teacher, he handed her the papers. She smiled and took them off him with a quick glance at the first sheet. Fraser looked at me disappointed, I understood his disappointment. We had put a lot of effort into that work and Fraser felt like he had really achieved something. Fraser went off into his area and I was told to go in the office for a quick chat. I hugged Fraser and told him it's going to be a good day baby.

In the office, they told me that they have contacted the local authority. The local authority has a service, a team who provide help for children on the autistic spectrum. They would come into school to observe Fraser and give staff training, tips and strategies to help. The service was very much overrun, with a long waiting list. However, they had managed to get an emergency appointment and they would be in tomorrow to observe Fraser. Is that ok, Mrs Stott? I agreed, any help was always appreciated.

I explained to Fraser what would be happening tomorrow in school; there will be strangers working with you, they're nice people and have come in to see why you are sometimes feeling upset. They have also come in to see if they can help your teachers as I don't think they understand autism very well! Fraser was happy, he said if they're here to help the teachers that's great as they need the help, not me! I chuckled at the way he viewed things. That's Fraser for you, stating the situation as he saw it and I wondered if he was actually right?

The plan was that the local authority would come into school on three separate occasions to observe and work with Fraser. The teachers would also receive training in autism and I was hoping again that things may improve.

The first observation went well. I say well, I wanted them to see how school were handling Fraser's difficulties. I was hoping that things wouldn't run smoothly so that we knew how things could improve, if that makes sense? The school priest had come into school that morning. The priest had asked all the children to line up as they made their way back from the library area. As he wandered down the corridor, Fraser was in a world of his own but not in a good place. He was in the middle of a busy queue and things were not running as planned. The arrival of the priest was unexpected and there was now a queue forming in front of the classroom as the children waited for a seat to listen to the priest. This waiting around was starting to frustrate Fraser. He was getting pushed around as the boys were shoving each other in the queue. The priest appeared at the classroom door and asked the children to walk into class. As he made this request, he grabbed Fraser's shoulders to direct him into the class. The priest had no idea about Fraser's condition but was he about to find out!

As soon as the priest put a firm hand on Fraser's

shoulder, our son's temper exploded. The pent up anxiety that had formed in that queue, along with his hypersensitivity to touch was like shaking a bottle of fizzy cola. Fraser turned on the priest immediately in what can only be described as the most inappropriate thing you could ever imagine saying to a member of the clergy:

"You're a big dick!", Fraser screamed at the ashen-faced priest.

"I'm not doing this, you're a dick head!", he bellowed at the man who stood there, mouth gaping.

Well as you can imagine, to say this was frowned upon is an understatement. Fraser was immediately escorted out of the class. In some ways, it was ideal for the people observing Fraser that day to witness this. At this stage, we had a feeling that there was something more than just autism at work. The autism-based strategies weren't having a huge impact on his behaviour and they needed to see this kind of thing to appreciate Fraser wasn't a run of the mill case. In fact, this incident which saddened me more than anything else, made me more determined to look deeper into what was happening. I wasn't convinced that Fraser had typical Asperger syndrome and something else was going on.

Chapter 11 – PDA and The Lightbulb Moment

I came home and switched on my laptop, search engine at the ready. Things weren't going well at all. The strategies school had been advised to try by the local authority team that had observed Fraser didn't really help. In fact, it seemed that they were having the opposite effect and making things ten times worse.

So there I sat on the sofa with my plumped cushions behind me and a warm cup of coffee by my side. I needed to understand how my son's mind was working, why was he so angry? He had a lovely home and a supportive family behind him. At school, things weren't good but things weren't always bad. As I scoured the web, reading countless articles and blogs, my mind was becoming overwhelmed with information overload. I wasn't exactly sure what I was trying to find but was searching for everything I could find about children who were anxious with extreme behaviour at school.

I was ready to give up for the evening. I was tired and felt that I hadn't found what I was looking for. I committed to reading one more article and it was as I read this article that my eyes started to widen. I began reading about a relatively little-known disorder called

Pathological Demand Avoidance (PDA) and it was describing every trait, nuance and behaviour we had seen in my son over these last few years. As I read on, my excitement grew. I had actually found something that described my Fraser and the article explained that there were ways to help improve things, strategies to use that were very successful.

It explained that PDA is part of the autistic spectrum and is an anxiety-driven condition seen in both children and adults. People with PDA experience a need to be in control of situations and feel compelled to avoid demands placed upon them by other people. In fact, the demand may not be explicit - it could be something such as a perceived expectation which most people do not even think twice about. Those with PDA will resist and avoid ordinary social expectations in their daily lives

In order to avoid these expectations, they may develop social strategies to help them deal with situations they were not comfortable with. For example, they may make up reasons for not participating in an event or activity. Whilst they may appear sociable on the surface, they could suffer excessive mood swings and be very impulse-driven. When those with PDA feel anxious, they can become driven by an uncontrollable need to take charge of their environment which may appear as controlling and dominating behaviour to others. This was also linked with problems controlling and regulating their emotions.

I sat there in awe – certain I had found the answer I had been so desperately seeking. I shouted down the stairs to Nigel in the kitchen… "Nigel, Nigel quick come up here, I need to show you something that I have found .. it's a double of Fraser!" He read the article and agreed that the article seemed to sum up some of Fraser's difficulties exactly.

It all fell into place.

When Fraser was at school he felt he was in an environment that was placing ever-changing demands on him. Whereas at home the demands were a lot less! The whole school day is packed with demands from start to finish:

- Fraser, wake up and get your uniform on for school!
- Line up in the queue before class
- Take your coat off and sit at your desk
- Walk slowly in the corridor
- Put your pack lunch box in the corner of the room
- Put your water bottle in your drawer
- Sit up straight!
- Raise your hand!
- Be quiet!

..all before 9.30am.

Imagine how many demands he had experienced by 3.15pm? Now all of this for a neurotypical child, whilst still demanding in some way, wouldn't be perceived the same way as a PDA child. A child with PDA who is generally extremely anxious would be experiencing an environment in which they felt they were losing control. Their fight or flight instincts would be heightened and ready to be invoked when things got too much.

I carried on reading the article and it spoke about strategies to help manage PDA. The main idea was to reduce demands and offer choices. It really was as simple as that. Once you learned this type of parenting or teaching, the anxiety in the child dropped and issues were minimal.

I was keen to learn more about the ways we could help Fraser and we followed the strategies on the PDA society website (**www.pdasociety.org.uk**) and I started to read every book I could find about PDA. The more I read the more I felt this sense of relief.

At first, it seemed like it was going to be a hard battle trying to figure out how I would change the way I worded things to Fraser .. and to reduce demands. I don't think we realise how many demands you can place on someone in one day. You will find that you can't eradicate all demands but if you can reduce them you will see massive changes in the home and school environment. Over time though, we found that all it really took was small adjustments to language.

Take bedtime for example. Instead of "It's time to get ready for bed now, Fraser", we would change the sentence to "Wow look at the time! Tell you what Fraser, get your pyjamas on and then you can have another 20 minutes playing on the Xbox before reading a book in bed".

Staying calm and neutral and using distraction works really well too. If I see that Fraser may be struggling in the morning to get changed for school, I'll simply talk to him about something as he puts his socks on. Likewise, instead of telling him to put his school clothes on they will already be laid on the bed so he can choose when to put his clothes on in the morning. To encourage him to put his clothes on we say that if he is able to do it now, he'll have time to do something he enjoys before setting off for school – be that reading a book, playing on his computer or watching part of a movie.

It took us some time as parents to get used to this approach. In a few weeks though, the change at home was astounding. To this day, our main approach is just to pre-warn him about anything and everything to avoid meltdowns:

- "Fraser, we need to go to the shops after the cinema, but we'll only be ten minutes"
- "Fraser, you'll have a different horse-riding teacher to the usual one today"
- "Fraser, you can have thirty more minutes watching TV and then it's time for bed"

Things seemed to calm a lot at home and we saw a big improvement. Things didn't seem as stressful and the house became more chilled, I think we had finally got the answer we were looking for.

I spent the next week researching as much as I could about PDA and joining more internet forums with other parents who also have PDA children. I have found that the best way to understand anything and get answers is speaking to those that are living with it every day - just like us.

I found a Facebook group for parents with PDA children and they held a regular meet-up. In fact, it was literally up the road from me. The parents would discuss different strategies and provide advice based on their own experiences. I still attend this group when I can to this day. I think it's so important to show others that they're not on their own and that there are other families just like us that are struggling and need support. It's such a shame that there are very few professional support groups available like this. Two years after Fraser was diagnosed with Asperger's we were offered a parenting course on the subject. The course offer came through two years too late and regardless, we needed something that was specific to PDA. There was a stark contrast between the autism strategies that were being implemented for Fraser by the local authority at school, and the PDA strategies we were starting to implement at home.

I had searched Amazon for books relating to PDA and even though they were few and far between, I was recommended an excellent book: Understanding Pathological Demand Avoidance in Children by Margaret Duncan, Ruth Fidler and Zara Healy Phil Christie. As soon as the book landed through the letterbox, I devoured every word, absorbing all the recommended strategies. Within a week of trialling these out at home, things were on the up and I felt confident to approach school with my findings. It was like I found a golden ticket.

The next morning, I walked into school with Fraser's hand clutched to the right of me and my book tightly tucked under my left arm. The headteacher was stood at the school gates greeting parents as they walked into school. I always prompted Fraser to try and say "good morning" in a happy voice when we arrived. I felt myself pacing up towards the head: "Good morning!" I exclaimed "I have found a book that explains everything! Can I come and see you once I have dropped Fraser off?" She looked at me in surprise and smiled, saying "Sure, I will see you soon". I dropped Fraser off at the class door and started to race back up to the gates where the head was still greeting parents.

"Did you have a good weekend, Mrs Stott?", I smiled and replied "Yes, I've been busy researching all about something called pathological demand avoidance". She looked at me confused and didn't have a clue what I was talking about. I took the book from under my arm and showed it to her. I started to blurt out everything about PDA, explaining how it was centred around a need for control and described Fraser's behaviour to a tee. I explained how just reducing some demands and rewording how you ask for things will make Fraser so much calmer and that the school will see a huge difference. She looked at me intrigued but not convinced. Later that day, I collected Fraser and was given back the book by his class teacher. Disheartened and not convinced it had been read, I reluctantly took it back. I looked at his class teacher in disappointment and asked her if she wanted to borrow it, I mentioned how handy it had become for us. She smiled and said to me that it would be useful, and she would have a read. I really hoped the book was read and it helped them manage Fraser.

The children in Fraser's class were still struggling to understand Fraser. I understood that some of the parents had started to complain to the school about his behaviour. At this stage, he was still prone to lashing out at classmates and he was a strong boy.

We knew that the school was under pressure to manage the situation and they suggested that maybe a letter to the other parents would help? I agreed, if they wanted to send out a letter then that would be fine and gave permission for this to be sent. We always tried to work with school each step of the way. They asked Fraser to write a piece to accompany the letter. When I saw what he had written, I cried:

The Letter from Fraser

My name is Fraser. I am 7 years old and you have been my friends for a long time.

Sometimes I think differently to other people and I am autistic.

There are lots of good things about me. I am good at dancing, swimming and singing and I have my own YouTube channel.

I find it hard trying to calm down and sometimes I say things that upset people or do things that upset people. I don't mean to but sometimes it makes people laugh or sometimes I find things hard to understand. I find school complicated.

I like being in year 3 and I have lots of friends. I was so happy when I was voted for school council because I thought I would never be on school council because I say no to everything all the time but it made me that happy that I screamed when I found out.

Thank you for all who try to help me and be my friend.

Fraser.

The letter was also attached with a list of symptoms detailing how hard it is for an Asperger's boy in school, in the hope that some of the parents may understand that we were all trying to deal with the situations that were arising as best as we could.

I received a few texts that evening from some understanding parents in class. This was a nice gesture when I had felt so pushed out for such a long time. I often thought to myself I wonder if they do realise how bad I feel for their children feeling scared of Fraser? He also has feelings too, how hurt he feels when the children run away from him in the playground or a child telling him that their mummy has said they can't play with him. The supportive and understanding texts meant a lot that night when the letter was sent out and I am still very grateful for them.

Things still weren't improving though and Fraser at this point was refusing to do any work in the class. I was concerned about his mental health, despite speaking to the school about PDA, a lot of the strategies being implemented were still non-PDA specific. I came home one day and sunk my head into my hands and burst in tears. I was at a low, no one knew how to manage my child. Fraser was coming home upset most evenings. Incident and restraints were very regular - to the extent that the teacher even felt awkward telling me on collection. Instead, she had offered to just give me a phone call, rather than being left there as the last parent standing on the playground, with Fraser pulling a sad face through the window with his thumb down. The calls were a better approach, but all day it put me in an anxious state, watching my phone for the school name to appear on the screen. I couldn't go far just in case I would be called into school when Fraser's meltdowns were bad and the school needed my help. Something had to give.

I started to investigate flexi-schooling, after all, Fraser was not learning much in school. He was spending most days at his desk outside the classroom or in the head's office after being restrained. The school didn't have funding for one to one support so often a teacher would sit with him on rotation. The teacher would help him for a few days then it would be someone different. The thing is, none of these teachers was used to dealing with an autistic PDA child. It seemed the teachers needed a break from Fraser as they couldn't teach him, and possibly his class peers also needed the break.

Fraser was in fight mode most days just waiting for the next teacher to grab him by the arm and lead him somewhere. Little did I know back then but there were a number of situations that evoked the basic human fight mode in Fraser. Much later on, we made a Subject Access Request to the school under the new General Data Protection Regulations (GDPR). This allowed us to obtain all records relating to Fraser's behaviour. Reading through this wealth of information, we discovered that in most incidents there was a trigger that caused Fraser to react. Fraser had been restrained regularly for around a month and things were getting out of hand. I didn't like the fact that adults were having to hold my son in such ways. He was a little eight-year-old boy, my little boy, I couldn't let this carry-on. How would this affect him later with other adults, would this make him completely lose trust in any adult if he thinks this is what teachers do? How will he ever want to learn or comply? Fraser needed love, he needed to be shown that he was liked and not treat like a naughty boy. One evening, after dwelling on this for a while my teary eyes looked at Nigel, "What are we going to do for our boy Nigel, this can't carry on we must be able to do something?"

I had come across flexi-schooling when it was mentioned on one of the Facebook groups I was a member of. Flexi-schooling is basically where a child is educated just part of the week in school and for the remainder of the week, they are educated at home. This is a legal approach as long as the headteacher and school governors accept the approach.

There is no requirement to follow the National Curriculum when educating a child at home either. Anything the parent deems educational for their child is acceptable so long as it does constitute some form of education.

In fact, the Education Act of 1996 includes a provision that applies to flexi-schooling. Rather than flexi-schooling being treated as an unauthorised absence, it can be defined as "leave" (in other words an *authorised absence*) so long as the head and governing body agree to it.

Section 444 (3) of the Act says:

The child shall not be taken to have failed to

attend regularly at the school by reason of his absence from the school:

(a) with leave

The term 'leave' is defined in Section 444(9) as:

"In this section 'leave', in relation to a school, means leave granted by any person authorised to do so by the governing body or proprietor of the school."

We decided the next day that we would email school and request a flexi-schooling approach. If the school agreed that they could effectively grant Fraser "leave" (i.e. an authorised absence) this would be a sufficient legal approach. I figured it was also an opportunity to keep him at his current school, at least for some of the week. At this point deregistering Fraser from school and taking him out for good was in the back of my mind too.

Almost immediately after sending the email, we were invited to a meeting to discuss flexi-schooling. I was nervous and worried that they would say no. I knew in the back of my mind that if they said no, I would have to seriously look at taking him out of school for good. I thought we didn't have any other option.

The head's office started to feel like a second home to me. I think I had been in there more than most staff that year, alongside Fraser. Nigel and I met with the headteacher and the executive headteacher. We discussed how we knew that things were going from bad to worse at school and we were very concerned about the frequency of restraints. We understood that staff and other children couldn't be placed at risk and we understood the reasons for restraining Fraser. However, it was happening too much, and we were concerned at this. We proposed that on a Thursday and a Friday we would educate Fraser at home, which left just three days at school. Their only concern was that Fraser may not want to come in on Monday because it may seem a longer weekend. I looked at them with exhausted eyes and said: "Please can we just give it a go? Surely it's worth a shot?" I promised them that I would try to get Fraser writing again. I explained that I wanted to do one to one activities with Fraser on Thursdays and then the Fridays would be spent at home working. They looked at me, nodded their heads and agreed that they would try the flexi-schooling and seemed happy to go along with this but would need to discuss it with the school governors because this was something that they had never done before.

A week later, we received the email to say that we were given permission to start flexi-schooling in the next half term. This was the point at which we started our second journey.

Chapter 12 – Flexi-Schooling

Fraser was good at telling me how he felt about things. To be honest, he has a great bond with me and opens up a lot. He always seemed very mature for his age and I have always been very honest with Fraser. I have felt I could be honest with Fraser as he is a bright boy and always seems to understand what I am telling him. Before diagnosis I would explain things to Fraser, exactly what was going to happen and pre-warn him about things. It makes me wonder how long I was putting all these strategies in place before we even knew about his diagnosis. I too am one for needing to know what's next and what is happening - maybe it was just in my nature to parent him this way?

Anyhow, I needed to speak to Fraser beforehand about this change to see if this was something that he wanted. I figured that this change impacted him, and he deserved to have a say in it. We spoke together about mummy doing two days of learning with him at home and how things could maybe improve at school this way. Fraser agreed that he still wanted to go to school but didn't like it when he had to sit in the office all the time and it was making him sad when the teachers kept holding him. Fraser was a little worried that he may miss out on work, but the fact was that he was missing work every day anyway.

I didn't want Fraser to think that being at home was just an excuse to sit and play on his Xbox or just a longer weekend. I wanted to prove to the school that teaching Fraser a different way, the way we had suggested all along, was more likely to keep him engaged. I had tried and tried to explain to school the strategies for dealing with PDA but very few of these had been adopted for teaching purposes.

Fraser was also keen to prove to the school that he could learn, so we decided that we needed a plan. Fraser would need to be in full control of what we learned if it was going to work. Our environment was going to be completely different from school. The learning activities we did on a Thursday would be more fun-based. Some of the activities we were doing on a weekend we would switch to a Thursday for this reason.

Swimming was becoming tricky on a Saturday as the pool environment was loud and Fraser was having difficulties concentrating. This was our last shot with swimming. We had been through three different swimming teachers, and then finally we had found one teacher who understood Fraser. He showed a great deal of compassion and was determined to engage Fraser in a way that made swimming fun. The feedback we'd had from other teachers was that he couldn't concentrate for long and became agitated. If the style of teaching was more direct and done in a way that didn't make it fun, there was no way Fraser would feel relaxed enough to learn. It was amazing when we finally found Jake who actually seemed to want to take on the challenge of bonding with Fraser and then teaching him to swim. The only problem was the busy pool, it was run by the university and was packed with students. Music played in the background and the pool would be very busy at times. I could tell that it was affecting Fraser to the brink of a sensory overload but he coped and managed. He was wearing earplugs and a headband to protect his ears due to his previous operation, which helped block out some of the noise, but then the next struggle was actually listening to Jake's instructions! Fraser would escape from the noise by ducking his head under the water and spent half the lesson that way. When Jake agreed that we could do lessons on a Thursday it was great news. The pool would be so much quieter and with that, we arranged lessons at 2pm each Thursday. Due to the environment change with the pool quieter, we slowly managed to take the headband away from Fraser as he was managing in a quieter environment. I witnessed Fraser being able to take more instructions, not being frustrated, and learning again!

The next activity we chose was horse riding. I read that the benefits for children with social-emotional disabilities come about due to the special relationship they develop with a horse. The horses at the RDA (Riding for the Disabled Association) are specifically chosen and trained to be gentle and calm. The unconditional, non-judgmental relationship between the horse and Fraser was just what he needed. Fraser's school experience had caused a breakdown in the way Fraser perceived people as being judgemental of him.

Equine therapy gives autistic children a sense of themselves, their bodies and increased contact and interaction with the surrounding world. Fraser's self-confidence seemed to be greatly increased after a few lessons. He formed a sense of competence by learning how to interact and work with the horse. As Fraser formed a good relationship with the horse I was hoping that this skill would transfer not only to his horse-riding teacher but also to the teachers at school.

The horse riding was great therapy for building relationships with those who teach Fraser in the future, but Fraser also has hypermobility which means that Fraser's joints are more flexible than what is considered normal. I was advised by the occupational therapist that core exercises would really help, so horse riding ticked the box for a PE lesson without Fraser even knowing this.

The physical benefits of horse riding are numerous. It relaxes tight muscles, increases balance, builds muscle strength, sharpens eye contact and hand coordination, improves fine motor coordination, helps gain a sense of self-body awareness, helps gain a sense of self-control and improves sensory integration.

We had a few horse-riding teachers before we found the right one. Again, tone of voice was tricky for Fraser, it still is now. You may be giving Fraser instructions in a very direct way and he will think you're shouting at him. So, we went through a couple of teachers before we found a male teacher/rider called Mike that understood Fraser. Well, he accepted that when Fraser suddenly went into Fortnite mode and spoke constantly about gaming that it was simply because Fraser was finding something too tricky. He sometimes babbled complete nonsense, but at no time did Mike once say, "What are you on about Fraser, we must carry on learning". Instead, we went with the lesson Fraser style!

If the lesson would get too much for Fraser, we would opt to go for a ride in the woods. Fraser would happily chat away with the teachers whilst on the horse, this alone was breath-taking - he was communicating with adults, not getting angry or frustrated, but socialising again.

Most lessons in this time period were spent on walks in the woods and that was fine with me, as long as he was happy. I needed my happy little boy back and seeing him laughing again and enjoying conversation was the exact thing he needed at that time.

Fridays were spent just me and him. We would have a busy Thursday and needed to put pen to paper if we could on a Friday. Fraser had stopped writing at school. School had given up on his writing and told us that he would use an iPad to record information to keep his anxiety low. I understood this, but whilst this was keeping his anxiety low it was just pushing him further and further away from what he was capable of doing. In the home setting, just me and him and with all my attention and support - I was sure we would get Fraser writing again.

If I wanted Fraser to do something, I would typically give him choices. However, the choices all consisted of things I wanted Fraser to achieve. This way, we would always have a productive outcome. I knew by asking Fraser if he could manage three lines of writing on a Friday, he would smash it. He was competitive and always wanted to prove he was better and could do better - this was my boy! I believe strongly this was one of the reasons why the large classroom didn't help Fraser's self-esteem. Fraser is a clever boy but he needs that little bit more processing time than others. This is a typical Asperger's trait. It isn't always easy for someone with Asperger's to listen to instructions and then comprehend their meaning as fast as others.

Fraser has a competitive nature. When he was amongst his class of thirty there were frequently situations where the other children grasped concepts and completed work much more quickly than him. He found this incredibly frustrating. In addition, he was overstimulated with the amount of noise, the pens scribbling, the boy next to him kicking the legs of his chair and the chatter around him. Add to that the fact that he is trying to get on top of the task himself but can't as he hasn't processed the instructions and can't concentrate enough to focus - it was then he would explode. It was uncontrollable, and he deeply regretted it when he had calmed down. Over time, this cycle damaged his self-esteem and any sense of self-worth.

When I told him about the writing, Fraser laughed at me and said "Only three lines? I can do more than three lines, I can do seven lines of writing!" I looked at Fraser with a shocked face "Really can you do seven lines?!! Wow, Fraser, that would be amazing, shall we give it a go?"

We started with creative writing, where I would let him decide what he wanted to write about. He would often choose to write about the activities we did the day before. The more that we did this, the more he wanted to write. He would often write an extra line to prove that he could write more than what was expected. Sometimes he would write one line, then walk away from it and circle round the room before thinking of his next sentence, then he would sit proudly back on his seat and write the sentence. For the third sentence, he may move position completely and spin on the kitchen stools and then write his third line. I smiled, I was happy. He was happy writing, he wasn't forced to sit at a table and a desk and conform like others, he did it his own way and it worked.

Don't get me wrong - we had our bad days, and not everything was plain sailing. Sometimes it was hard to teach Fraser. It was January 2018, a Monday morning, and the snow was coming down deep. I checked the school's website and it was expected for pupils to still attempt the journey. We lived a fifteen-minute drive from school but that morning it took an hour and a half to get even close to the school. The traffic was bad, and I had two school runs to do. First was for my eldest son which was only a three-minute drive from Fraser's school. We attempted to drive up the hill towards Tyler's school, but the wheels were spinning, it was scary and the snow was still falling. It was due to carry on falling all day. I made the decision to turn around, you can imagine both boys were happy that we were driving back home. When we got home I thought it would be a good idea to do some work with Fraser, after all, it was still a school day. I had a book that we would use to put in all the work that we had achieved at home.

When we got back home, the boys went outside to start building snowmen, everything that you would do on a snowy day. Fraser bounded through the door with bright red cheeks after thirty minutes saying he'd had enough. Tyler wasn't helping him enough and they were starting to have brotherly differences on who was collecting the right amount of snow. I helped take off his wellies and got him dry. I grabbed some logs for the wood burner and mentioned to Fraser how we could carry on doing the work we were doing from last week.

Bang! Tears immediately flowed as Fraser exclaimed: "Why do I have to do work?" I said, "Well it's still a school day and surely we could do a little extra?" Fraser looked at me confused but agreed he would give it a go. Within five minutes of starting to write the first sentence we started hearing the excuses "My hand is hurting, I feel sick, I have a headache" these were things that Fraser would say if he wanted to get out of the demand being given but he also experiences a sick feeling when his anxiety is rising. I pushed it still and didn't listen "Let's get to your five lines and we will call it a day", I said calmly.

"You stupid dumb fucking idiot I don't want to!", he screamed at me. He then repeated it again right up to my face. I was shocked, really shocked. He had never sworn at me or got this angry at me before, it hurt really bad. I held back my tears and told Fraser "Mummy needs some time on her own. Mummy is angry right now and I am not happy about what you have just called me, you will not be going to horse riding this week either". I ran upstairs to my bedroom, shut the door and crouched in a ball next to the door and burst in tears. I wondered if I had completely just blown it. Fraser was doing so well and I pushed him and didn't listen to him. I did exactly the things I shouldn't have done, how could I have been so stupid? I then went on further to take something away from him and it really wasn't his fault. Yes, Fraser shouldn't be talking to me in that manner but how could I, his parent, fall in the trap of treating him the same way that those who didn't understand him treated him? Everyone makes mistakes. I took a deep breath and walked back down the stairs. Fraser was sat at the table, with tears in his eyes. He had a pencil in one hand and his writing book in front of him. He looked at me and cried, he said "I am so so so sorry mummy. Look, I've done 8 lines for you". I hugged him tightly. "You shouldn't be sorry Fraser. Mummy should be sorry because I didn't listen to you". Fraser was trying to catch his breath from sobbing and said "…but mummy it's not a home education today, it's not Friday. I shouldn't be doing work, Tyler isn't doing work right now, he doesn't have to sit and do homework. He's watching TV. I don't know why I have to be made to be different on a snow day?" Fraser was so right. As much as you want to push your child when you feel they're turning a corner and doing so well, you must listen carefully to when they give you the warning signs of anxiety building. Fraser also sees the world very black and white! Monday was not a home education day.

We had our ups and downs and I began to learn a lot about Fraser from our home ed days. I learnt that Fraser needed space to move around. Fraser needed to set his own boundaries to keep his anxiety levels low, he would then raise the bar himself to impress me. I learnt that Fraser needed extra support just as I was giving him. He sometimes needed me by his side but sometimes he was happy to get on with things his own way whilst I managed to run around the house with the hoover, or even better, grab a cup of coffee! Fraser needed to feel like he was achieving again and that he had no competition to keep his anxiety low and do things on his terms. I would set him something that I knew was easy/achievable, but Fraser would want to please and rise above it. I learnt to listen to Fraser when he said that he was starting to feel poorly. I learnt to divide work into small chunks and break it up if I knew that his anxiety was rising. When I saw him becoming anxious we could get a drink or go for a walk. I learnt that he wasn't a frustrated boy at home or even outside the home and any form of frustration was normally a way of Fraser communicating his struggles. He didn't have the maturity to explain that there was too much sensory overload! Every time Fraser got angry or frustrated there was always a reason behind it.

We had great fun learning, in a way I am glad I had the opportunity to spend time with Fraser more, as our bond strengthened. We visited zoos and did projects on the animals, we even had great fun planning our Disney trip by drawing maps showing the waiting time for rides and throwing maths in there! It was great for Fraser to plan his holiday also as he felt in complete control of our vacation that we had planned later in the year. I was even lucky enough to get in touch with my old friend Sarah who is now a scientist for a large hospital in the breast cancer unit. We visited the lab and did some amazing science experiments! I felt the opportunities and learning that we did on our Thursdays and Fridays were more than what he had managed at school. I filled his book with pages of work that Fraser had produced, he was even writing full pages himself with no anxiety building up. Every Friday evening, I would write a little report on what changes we made to help Fraser over those two days and what worked and what didn't work. On Monday, Tuesday and Wednesday things would go a little smoother at school. I didn't receive any feedback from my reports but all I could still do was to let them know what was working. It seemed they did a good job of telling me what wasn't working whilst I did a great job of telling them what was working!

I decided that I would start my own Facebook group and document our journey. There seemed to be a lot of groups for families with autistic children but there didn't seem to be many groups discussing PDA or at least documenting a child's progress with PDA. I figured that if I had somewhere to document everything, I could always fall back on this as my evidence of what we had been doing, or even as a diary to remember different stages of Fraser's development. We had our notebook but sometimes videos captured our moments. The page helped me the most by connecting me to a group of supportive people together going through the same situations as us. It's great not to feel on your own and know that others are going through the same experience. I still run this group and if you're reading this I am guessing you have a child similar or going through a similar process to us, so pop along to **www.facebook.com/alienplanet**

We were lucky enough to meet some amazing people, and in our journey of flexi-schooling met some wonderful parents that did and are doing an amazing job home-schooling their children. Not only did flexi-schooling help Fraser with his learning again, but Fraser was also actually making friends! Real friends, friends just like him that hadn't been accepted at school, made to feel like the odd one out, parents who made the decision to take their children out of education before there was too much damage. We were very lucky to meet one lady who has become a close friend. She had two boys out of school at the time who came to play with Fraser, facing similar battles as ourselves. The time that Fraser spent playing with her boys was invaluable, it made Fraser feel wanted again. For once we had friends that wanted to come and play and be in Fraser's company rather than to be told to stay away from him. I also met another wonderful lady with three children on the spectrum currently home educating. She lives in Doncaster, so it's hard to arrange meet-ups as often, however she encouraged her children to write to Fraser and he would do the same back. All these children aren't strange or difficult, they're children that just need understanding, patience and to be allowed to blossom.

When you flexi-school your child, it's sometimes easy for others to look down on this as a negative thing. They may think that you must have it all because instead of working, you get to spend time at home with your child. You may also be criticised for depriving your child of the opportunity to socialise with other children. For parents, flexi-schooling involves a lot of ·sacrifices. It's very difficult to devote time to yourself and taking on the role of a teacher, when you are untrained and finding your way is difficult. Fraser socialised with more people during those two days of home-schooling than he ever did at school. We were creating a whole new circle of friends and it was a breath of fresh air for Fraser. I knew that no-one could understand unless they were going through this and when I heard comments that seemed critical of what I was doing, I simply ignored them. I knew that even just providing these two days for him would stop him from entering into a low depressive state. Fraser's self-esteem was the lowest that I had ever seen it. He was certainly not socialising at school, sat outside in the hallway at his desk or in the head's office.

Flexi-schooling certainly had its benefits in getting him learning again, making friends, socialising, and boosting his confidence.

The new term came and we had agreed to meet with the school to discuss the home-schooling situation. To my surprise, the headteacher looked at me and asked me for ideas on what Fraser would like to learn at school. I couldn't help but laugh. I said, "I can't tell you what I'm going to do with Fraser in case you use my ideas and I have nothing left for home-schooling!" I explained that I didn't have time to plan out Fraser's work for school, I wasn't a teacher. To be fair, each week I went with the flow, there were so many ideas that we could do but it all depended on how Fraser felt that day that influenced in which order we would do work. As long as you were giving Fraser choices, anything would work really.

In further conversations with the school, they indicated that they were still struggling to provide Fraser what he needed. Flexi-schooling certainly was giving everyone a break and maybe, just maybe, would I like to do more flexi-schooling days? I had to go away and think about this, were they telling me they couldn't cope? If they couldn't cope what were they expecting to do? Were they waiting for an opportunity to be able to exclude Fraser? At this point, I thought that maybe the school were going through a process to try and get Fraser into a school that was better catered for his needs. They acknowledged that this whole situation was a very new thing for them and I knew that just finding the resources to cater for things like one to one support was difficult. They had managed to secure some additional funding but it wasn't a huge amount. I think both the school and I knew that that, deep down, Fraser needed a different type of environment. I can't fault the school for everything they did – they never gave up and I am grateful for that. The thing is, there is only so much they could do.

Chapter 13 - Dealing with the Effect and not the Cause

I thought a lot. It was going around in my head over and over why he was not coping at all in the mainstream environment. He could cope at concerts and other busy places with me. It was just the learning. There was always a reason behind Fraser's behaviour, but the teachers were too overstretched to have the time to assess Fraser in this level of detail.

The problem was, that at school, the *effect* of Fraser's behaviour was being addressed rather than the *cause*. Any disruption from him would be met with some kind of punishment or sanction.

It had been mentioned to me by a teacher how they had previously taught autistic children at school. However, they remarked how our son was on a different level and they just hadn't seen this before. The school really didn't know what to do, and despite their best efforts to accommodate all manner of reasonable adjustments, specialist help was needed.

We must have spent hours and hours in the school office discussing target sheets and strategies, but none of these were PDA strategies. In a meeting with the local authority, I raised a point on how PDA strategies work, but they didn't seem to want to listen. Fraser hadn't received his private diagnosis of PDA back then and the local authority attitude to PDA was patchy and sporadic. When we did eventually get the private diagnosis of PDA, it helped bring the issue to the table. Even though we were reminded that PDA wasn't formally recognised on numerous occasions by the local authority, they did seem more willing to give it some acknowledgement with a diagnosis.

Over the months, I realised that I needed to really explore the reasons that sat behind Fraser's behaviour. It was so easy to get distracted by "the process" – getting a diagnosis, helping your child through school, and home-schooling that the days would fly by without the opportunity to really think about things. Thinking outside the box requires space for contemplation.

Some of the things that Fraser was attempting at school in order to help him were having the opposite effect. A lot of the strategies were designed to identify when Fraser had been a "good boy" or a "bad boy". We had the green face, orange face and red face system that would indicate how his behaviour had been perceived. This behaviour chart approach would grade Fraser's behaviour throughout the day. Every time Fraser did something that school didn't want him to do he would get a red face on the chart. If things went well he would receive a green face and if things went ok it was an orange face. He was given targets such as using safe calm hands 80% of the time or not shouting out in class 60% of the time. These were attempts to stifle his behaviour and not address the root cause of it.

I did wonder whether Fraser's lagging skills could be at the heart of some of the behaviour. Lagging skills are underdeveloped skills in children which hinder their ability to deal with a situation.

If left, lagging skills can be an unsolved yet significant problem. However, it was easier for people to just blame the autism, "It must be his autism", they would say in response to anything they didn't understand.

Fraser had difficulty in managing his emotional response to frustration and he struggles to think rationally. This is the reason he would shout out in class. I began to wonder if maybe we could offer more support to help him understand his emotions? A big red face on a sheet confirmed to Fraser that he had done something wrong but told him nothing about how to manage it next time. Each red face given was a little piece of self-esteem taken. As you can imagine we got a lot of red faces on lots of slips of paper. These sheets of paper would be given to Fraser to hand over to me when I picked him up in the afternoon. I learnt quickly that these sheets of paper meant nothing to us and I made that clear to him. If he thought that I may be disappointed or angry with him on collection, his anxiety levels would rise even higher at school. I was trying my best to reduce his anxiety, not heighten it. Besides, I wasn't disappointed or angry with him at all. I knew he didn't want any of this, no more than anyone else. You could see that he was upset handing me the paper with a sense of disappointment, but if he had a bad day I would just explain to him that it wasn't his fault. I held his hand tight and screwed the sheet up in a tight ball with my other hand. We would then walk out of the school gates with my head held high, and once back at the car I'd give him a big cuddle. He would ask me in the car "Mummy are you mad with me?" I would look at him and smile back and reassure him that mummy is not mad and we will go home and have a lovely evening. Tomorrow is always a new day at school.

I understood the teacher didn't have time to work out reasons for the unsolved problems that my son was having each day. I know lots of parents with children awaiting diagnosis were encouraged to go on parenting courses as though the parents may be the ones that were aggravating the behaviour in their children. No-one suggested this to us but I did wonder if people thought our parenting was the cause of some of these problems. Everyone has busy jobs but solving the problems would take less time than leaving it unsolved. The exhausted teacher that has thirty children to teach doesn't have time to think about the cause, neither does anyone else in school I guess – it was obvious to us that examining the cause rather than managing the effect was never going to happen in mainstream school.

Based on discussions with other parents and professionals, I believe that a lot of mainstream primary schools take the same approach to children with challenging behaviours. They look at things on the surface. They deal with the triggers that are very obvious and implement extreme, perhaps archaic measure to address them. For example, Fraser worked on a desk outside of the classroom a lot of the time. This stopped him from being triggered by the noise or disorder of the class but at the same time ostracised him socially. Surely, focusing on the cause of the problem in order to help and support that child long term was more important than the green smiley faces they had on that sheet of paper? The targets in the IEP were also meaningless. They were a pipe dream based on how they wanted my child to behave with absolutely nothing in place to truly understand what was going on in his head. Can mainstream schools really be expected to provide this level of support? I don't think they can under the current system.

Children do well if they can – if they can't, adults need to step in to figure out what's getting in the way so they can help.

- Identifying the unsolved problem or lagging skill;
- Using different approaches to teach the child;
- Working together as parents and teachers;
- Solving problems with your child rather than demanding that your child must change.

I am strongly of the belief that approaches to supporting children with special educational needs should change, rather than expecting a child to change. I learnt this from a very genuine and wonderful lady called Yvonne Newbold, who ran another Facebook group (The SEND VCB Project).

I had read a lot of the posts by Yvonne and I believe this was the moment when the penny dropped for us that Fraser just wasn't in the right environment. The environment would never change, and neither would he whilst he was there.

Chapter 14 – Specialist vs. Mainstream Provision

Fraser was and is a clever little boy. As parents, we thought that Fraser would sail through mainstream school. In the early days we believed that if we could get some extra support after his diagnosis, he would get through it. But the more and more I learnt how Fraser *could* thrive, I realised it wasn't going to be in a class of thirty children. In fact, I believed that even half of that number would still prove tricky.

Fraser was competitive amongst groups of children. He had it in his head that he had to be the best at everything. In a large class, this was always going to give way to frustration. Fraser struggled hugely with the noise, he found that he could no longer concentrate or block out background noise. I offered Fraser the choice to wear ear defenders, but he was adamant he wanted to fit in with his peers. He didn't want to look different, it was damaging to his self-esteem and he longed to just fit in and be like everyone else.

Fraser was struggling at lunchtimes as the school hall with two hundred and eighty pupils inside would tip him over the edge. The smells of other foods made him gag, the smell of yoghurt he found particularly tormenting.

Fraser needed time to understand his schoolwork, it needed to be broken up into tasks. His processing time was slower than others and he needed that extra time to absorb instructions.

Fraser longed for friends, but he needed help to form friendships and to keep them. It seemed that every chance he had to make friends at school had been blown away. He was seen as the naughty or strange kid to his peers and he knew that, he longed to be the same as other boys in the school.

Where would he go? Where would he fit in? We ruled out mainstream as he hadn't coped there for the last four years. We considered a mainstream setting with a hub or base attached to the school. There seemed to be a wide selection of these, but we realised that Fraser would only be back in the same position that he was now. He would have a base or hub to access learning and then, when the school would think that he was coping, would he be encouraged to access their mainstream environment? We knew that Fraser would feel singled out, he wanted nothing more than to be a boy, a cool boy, not the boy that has autism and is different.

Our next option was to look at specialist schools. I figured that if we could find a school for Fraser that had other Asperger's boys he would feel accepted. There was more of a possibility that he could access the different therapies he required, such as improving his social and communication skills, along with speech and language support in a smaller and specialist setting.

I began to look at all the specialist settings in the area, but came across one hurdle, all specialist settings required an Education and Health Care Plan

(EHCP) to be in place.

An EHCP is a legal document that is a pre-requisite for children attending most specialist schools. It lays out a child's special educational needs (SEN) and how these will be addressed. Not all children with SEN require an EHCP and the process to get one can be long and arduous. This is because the local authority takes on certain legal obligations when a child has an EHCP and they don't get handed out easily.

We realised it wasn't just as simple as moving Fraser to a different school. This was going to be another hurdle that we faced but we didn't realise how draining that process was going to be.

Another school meeting was arranged. Nigel and I sat in what seemed, at this stage, to be our personal chairs in that room. We explained that whilst we appreciated the school were trying to do everything possible we just couldn't see how it was going to get better. I wasn't in a position to take on more flexi-school days. Also, I wasn't a teacher so that wasn't going to be a way forward. The school hadn't heard of PDA and didn't seem keen to learn about it in detail, so in my eyes his anxiety was always going to be at a high. The mainstream school environment was placing too many demands on him and we knew that it had come to the end of the line.

When we explained all this to the school, there did seem to be a sense of relief amongst the school representatives present in that meeting. I think they were unsure what this meeting was going to be about and were they worried that they could not meet our expectations? I explained that as parents, we believe that Fraser will thrive once again but in a smaller setting - a specialist setting. We explained that Fraser, however, would need an EHCP, everyone in that room was still nodding their heads at us. They said, "That will be fine, just let us know what we need to do and we will get one!"

If only it was that easy. We walked away that afternoon feeling relieved that we had a plan. That evening I went home and emailed the school about what we had discussed. I had learnt always to leave a paper trail after each meeting, outlining what was discussed just in case I ever needed to clarify who had said what and when.

The next day I bumped into the headteacher who wanted a quick word. She mentioned that she was looking into applying for Fraser's EHCP but she warned me that it may be rejected. She explained to me that children who receive an EHCP have to be severely behind in their work - like two to three years behind. Fraser was currently only a year behind even though he had not been in the class much during year three. She explained that her gut instinct was that we wouldn't be able to get one, but if this is something I wished for her to go ahead and do then she would.

I felt saddened by the lack of confidence, where would we end up without an EHCP? Would Fraser eventually get permanently excluded from school?

Flexi-schooling was going well, and I even thought about removing Fraser from the roll and home-schooling him permanently. I was no teacher but figured that as long as Fraser was happy that was all that counted. We could learn the basics and I could even get a tutor for maths and English. I was concerned about what would happen if we couldn't get the right school for Fraser. Nigel would tell me "what's the worst that can happen – he'll just stay at home and learn here". I agreed.

As always, we spoke to Fraser about what he wanted. Fraser has a strong personality and if we were going to put him somewhere that he didn't feel entirely comfortable, the whole process would be pointless. He needed to be part of this.

As always, we gave Fraser choices. We explained that we could try to make things work at his current school for longer, to which he shook his head to indicate that wasn't an option. We explained that we could look for another school that had children just like him? Fraser smiled and nodded. The last option we gave him was that if he really wanted to, he could stay at home with mummy and we will get teachers to come to our home. It would be like our flexi-schooling days. Fraser quickly gave me his view on flexi-schooling, he said, "Mummy - I enjoy our days but I just want to go to a school and be like other boys at school. I want to be around friends", at this point he burst into tears. I felt bad, I maybe shouldn't have asked him, but I needed to know what he wanted. I would have hated it if I pushed him into an environment that he didn't want to be in. Possibly, his upset was because he was a young child and worried. Asperger's children don't often cope with change, and this was going to be a big change for him. I always felt Fraser had a mature head and I knew he needed to know what was happening, if he didn't it would cause more anxiety. Fraser needed to be involved each step of the way. However, I hadn't properly considered how Fraser would react to this. I do believe it made things worse for the school as Fraser doesn't have a filter. Fraser walked into school the next morning telling all his class friends that he was leaving. He was going to a school where they understood more about autism and that he was too clever for this school. Fraser told teachers that he was going to another school, he wasn't sure which one just yet but mummy is finding another one for me.

That evening I had to have another little chat with Fraser, we had to explain the time frame, it wasn't going to happen straight away. Mummy and Daddy have to get a document called an EHCP, we explained that this would tell his next school all about him and all the teachers would read it and understand him better. I explained that when Fraser started his current school, they didn't have this and didn't know that he needed his work cut into chunks, school didn't know that he may need a quieter place to eat his dinner or even little things such as needing a calm place to go if he felt the noise was too much. No one knew anything, not even mummy and daddy who knew him the best. I explained that we all had to learn this, school needed time to get a few people in to observe him and write reports. These reports would help to write this important document all about him for his next school. It may take about half a year before we can even start to look at another school which means that he had to be patient. Things will happen, but they won't happen tomorrow.

Fraser kind of understood this, I don't think he quite understood the timescale of half a year and possibly still thought it was like the end of the month or something.

I started my search for schools which prompted me to ask advice on our local autism Facebook group. To my dismay, when I asked about specialist schools for bright children in the local area, I was told quite simply that they didn't exist. If we wanted a specialist school where our boy would be given opportunities to academically thrive and achieve, we would need to look at independent schools outside of the local authority area. The support charity, SCOPE, had a service that helped parents with the EHCP process, and I approached them for assistance. Unfortunately, I believe this specific service that helped us has now closed, but there are charities out there that are listed at the end of this book. A kind and knowledgeable lady at SCOPE called Janine helped us. She sent me over a list of all the specialist schools in our area and then a list of independent schools that were outside the local authority area. Before looking at the independent schools, I thought it was best to review the local authority schools first. I knew that the local authority would be keen to put Fraser in a school within the area before considering an independent out of authority provision. The cost of independent specialist schools can be high and the local authority would only use such a school as a last resort. For this reason, I needed to do some detailed research. It's a reality that money drives much of the special educational needs system and the independent out of authority schools would be a significant overhead for the local authority. I Googled each school and made a note of the ones that I thought may be suitable. I managed to find a few schools and added them to my list, although it seemed that a few of these schools had bases which were then attached to the mainstream part. A "base" may simply be a classroom for SEN children within a mainstream school. They may then attend some lessons in mainstream classrooms.

We had just come out of a difficult mainstream experience, but I figured out that I should go and view these schools regardless. Maybe my thoughts would be different if I went to view them? I booked an appointment to view two local schools close by to me. One was wonderful – the staff were dedicated and provided an amazing level of care for the children there. However, it wasn't geared up for children that were academically very capable, the facilities were great but more geared towards severely disabled children. The classroom had children functioning at such a different level, he wouldn't be able to form a good peer friendship group.

The next school I visited was the type of school that was mainstream but had a special educational needs base. Upon arrival we were told immediately that the whole aim of a placement there would be for Fraser to eventually join the mainstream environment. Immediately, I knew this was a no go. Fraser had struggled for too long in the mainstream environment, I was searching for a small school that would understand and support his sensory profile. I wanted him to be around children like him so that he didn't get bullied and feel like the odd one out again. I didn't want to force him into an environment where he would be compelled to cope – no, we wanted Fraser to thrive. We were ushered into the base classroom at the school. The base was a pleasant little room with around six children. All the children greeted myself and my husband and they seemed fairly happy. I asked the teacher "Where do the children go when they are in crisis? Do they have an area to calm?" To my dismay, she replied "No, we don't have anywhere in particular … though the toilet is just through that door (she pointed to a door behind us).. the kids go in there, have a good scream and then come back".

My heart sank. I tried to pick my jaw up from the floor and looked at my husband who also appeared astounded by the remark. Enough was enough. We headed on to the next local authority school...

On our way there, we drove down a long driveway before the school popped into sight. What struck me first was the high prison-like security fence that circled the perimeter of the building. We drove up to a large electric gate that loomed over us. We pressed the buzzer to announce ourselves and watched as the gate slid open to make way for our car to enter. We walked into reception and signed our names in the visitor book. A member of staff greeted us and announced that she would be showing us around the school. She quickly warned us that when we walked around the school, there may be some children in crisis and we may hear some swearing. As we walked around we saw staff trying to do their best in the situation that they were in. Some children were angry, very angry. One boy walked past us kicking the walls, then we saw another walking down the corridor and into the office as it seemed his finger had been badly cut. He was shouting and swearing (I possibly would have been if I had done the same to my finger!)

We walked past some small cell-like box rooms. They were about the size of a cupboard with nothing in them apart from a padded seat and walls. The rooms had doors on them and a little window. I asked about these rooms, is this where children go in crisis to calm down? The staff member told us that we were right, this is where children go when in crisis. She explained that the rooms are very plain because they don't want children to stay there for long and that the doors were never shut. It did leave me wondering though, why the doors were put there in the first place? This school clearly didn't strike us as they type of environment in which Fraser would thrive. Our search continued.

Schools in our local area weren't looking promising for us. Don't get me wrong, there were some amazing schools that were doing a fantastic job with the children there. The staff were dedicated, and the children were getting the best care for their needs. The issue was that the children in the schools had such an array of different challenges and disabilities. Fraser had Asperger's and PDA. He needed a very specific type of support and we just hadn't found that yet.

My search for an out of authority independent school began and I quickly came across a school that I thought was ideal. The school was for boys, boys that were high functioning Asperger's and the school ethos fitted Fraser's profile. They were keen to not use restraint in times of crisis and had a hands-off policy. The school was small with sixty pupils on roll and with class sizes of five or less. This sounded perfect and I knew immediately that I needed to book a visit. The journey from home took around fifty minutes but if it could be the right school where Fraser would learn and thrive, then so be it!

I was really excited about this visit. After researching other out of area schools, nowhere seemed to have a patch on this school. On a bright July day, my husband and I took the scenic drive which was countryside for the majority of the journey. Before long, the sat nav indicated we were here and we turned right to drive down a long driveway. As the stately-home-style towers of the school came into view, I was reminded of Hogwarts from the Harry Potter movies. The building was old and very quiet, completely different from what we had seen before. There were no high fences - just a sense of a calm that fell over the place. We made our way to reception, signed in and waited to see the head.

I was very impressed by the headteacher. He explained to us about his role there and gave us an example of how he operated. He described how sometimes, some boys would sit under the table in the classroom. As head of this school, he explained, it wasn't his job to shout at the boy and demand he gets out from under the desk. No, it was his job to sit under the desk with the boy and find out why he was there. The conversation went well, the head was a nice guy, seemed on our level, and understood our situation. The conversation led to Fraser's age. Fraser was too young to start at the school as he was seven at the time and nearly eight but he wouldn't be able to start school until he was nine years old. The head explained to us that they have an assessment process which Fraser would need to go through to determine whether the school would be suitable for him. He also emphasised that we should come back to him once we have an EHCP as they could only accept boys who already held an EHCP.

We walked out of the school gates, looked at each other and smiled. As soon as I got in the car my smile beamed further - I had found the school I needed but

… what would we do in the meantime? He needed to be nine years old, we would have a year and a half to wait before we could start the application process and Fraser needed somewhere soon? Maybe we just had to be patient and wait? I couldn't think of any other ideas. It would be wrong to move Fraser for a year into a school that wasn't right for him only to then move him again. We lamented that we would just have to be patient and wait!

Chapter 15 - The EHCP

To obtain an EHCP you need to be able to demonstrate that your child has additional needs and requires more support than is currently available to them in their existing setting. Fraser had his IEP but we felt that the support he had was proving inadequate and the school had said to us on more than one occasion that they didn't feel they could meet Fraser's needs despite all the efforts they were making.

We had our last appointment with the specialist local authority autism agency. They had once again been into school to suggest ideas and strategies. We emphasised yet again that Fraser works well with PDA strategies rather than other autism strategies. We felt that a mainstream school wasn't suitable for Fraser and we had found a school out of authority, however, we need the EHCP to be able to get a place. We told this to the lady who had come into see Fraser and trying to manage our expectations, she told us "This school is a very difficult school to get into. Their fees are high, and it may be a battle to get your child in there. I would be mindful that this may not happen".

I left that meeting even more determined. Fraser had the diagnosis of Asperger's, and there were boys in that school that are the same as my son. They got a place so why couldn't we? Why wasn't our child deserving of a place also? But again, the age barrier was an issue. I guessed if we got the EHCP and plodded along at his current mainstream school it would all fall into place.

Nigel and I were committed to getting a place for Fraser and decided that we may need some legal help to obtain an EHCP. I guess a few people had said things that worried us and we thought that getting an EHCP agreed by the LA may be tricky, after all, we were told that Fraser didn't seem behind enough educationally.

Obtaining an EHCP is a multi-step process. The rules for this process are set out in the Children and Families Act 2014. To be honest, the law provides a lot of protections for families, and places strict rules on what a local authority can and can't do during this process. The first step in obtaining an EHCP is for the parents, child or school to approach the local authority and request an EHCP needs assessment. This is where the local authority assesses whether they think an EHCP is actually needed for the child. We had been advised by many parents that our local authority had turned down children for an EHCP at this first hurdle. We knew, therefore, it was important to come out fighting from the outset and not take anything for granted.

We contacted a local firm of solicitors and spoke to an EHCP specialist there. He told us that we could pay a one-off fee of £600 to put all Fraser's evidence together and they would then approach the LA, highlighting their legal obligation to assess Fraser for an EHCP. The law states that a local authority must consider two things when determining whether or not to carry out an EHCP needs assessment:

- Firstly, they must determine whether the child or young person has or may have special educational needs ("SEN"); and
- Secondly, whether the child may need special educational provision to be made through an EHC plan.

If the answer to both of these questions is yes, then the local authority must carry out an EHC needs assessment.

The solicitor then advised us that fighting for an EHCP could be a lengthy process which may end up at a tribunal. Therefore, we also had the option to pay a one-off fee of £7000 that would cover the costs of fighting the LA if they refused an EHCP at any point. We decided we would find the £600 for submitting the evidence and a letter and see how we went from there. Nigel is a clever man and felt confident that he could fight the LA if we needed to. He didn't feel the need for us to go in debt, though I was desperate to ensure all bases were covered and begged him to put the £7000 on a card and let the solicitor do it for us if it came to it. I explained to Nigel that he had a busy job and if we needed to, he wouldn't have time to take this on, but he asked me to trust him. "Katie, you must trust me when I say I can do it, I will do it".

School at this point had submitted the first part of the EHCP assessment request form to say they wanted Fraser to be assessed for an EHCP. The process differs from area to area, but our LA had forms that could be submitted by schools, parents, and the child, to request an EHCP assessment. Some areas don't really have a formal process and require a letter to be written. We received some information about the EHCP assessment request process from the LA and the next step after submitting the initial forms would see us attend a Multi-Agency Panel (MAP) meeting. This is when the school, parents and local authority professionals are invited to meet and discuss aspects of the assessment application. The LA examine the evidence submitted and determine at the meeting whether they should proceed to an EHCP assessment. I felt confident, if they said no then we would appeal and fight again, it was the start of the journey, a new journey for Fraser.

MAP day came and I felt sick. My nerves were on edge but I needed to put across my confident fighting mum persona that I had been using all along in this journey so far. We met with our school SENCO just before the meeting was due to start and we all went in together. She also looked nervous as this was her first time attending a MAP meeting in this context. I think she was just as keen to get what we wanted as us.

We took our seats and sat down. There were five professionals from the local authority in the room. Besides the lady chairing the meeting, there were two educational psychologists and two local authority caseworkers. At one end of the room was a screen with notes about Fraser displayed. On-screen, they brought up a PowerPoint presentation we had submitted as part of our parents' section of the EHCP assessment application. We had included photos of Fraser as I believed seeing the child we were talking about meant it became a little more personal than just reading a name from a sheet of paper. The SENCO did an amazing job and did pretty much all the talking about how the school were being challenged daily and how Fraser needed a setting in which he would thrive once again. Nigel and I seemed to lose our words in that meeting, I guess I was too scared to speak in case I put my foot in it. I knew the meeting was important and if I said the wrong thing, I would never have forgiven myself. However, I knew Nigel was clever and I was hoping he would have some input, but we both seemed to freeze. Maybe we had underestimated the level of scrutiny they were putting into this. At the end of the meeting, we were asked as parents why we wanted the EHCP. The only right answer I knew here was to explain that I was looking at a specialist setting and I knew we needed the EHCP to be able to get admission. At that point, the Chair asked each of the local authority professionals in the room whether they thought they should proceed to an EHCP assessment by answering yes or no. Our worry began to dissipate as in turn, each professional agreed that an assessment should proceed. The only person who wasn't sure was the chairperson herself who announced that she was on the fence but would allow the assessment to proceed given everyone else had supported it.

The panel mentioned, that as part of the assessment, there needed to be further reports completed to ensure all the information they had was complete and up to date. The assessment is conducted to determine whether an EHCP is actually needed for the child. To make this decision, the LA review reports written by specialists. A local authority Educational Psychologist would be coming into school to assess Fraser, and the LA said that they would also consult with CAMHS and their own autism specialists for additional evidence. As parents, we could approach other professionals and obtain our own reports.

The LA would then review all the reports that had been collated and make a decision as to whether they would issue an EHCP or not. At this stage, it was important not to sit back and leave the LA to gather their own professional reports. We had an opportunity to approach other professionals and obtain our own reports. I knew that we needed input from every professional that had been involved with Fraser. I needed as many reports as possible to create a true image of Fraser so that when it came to these documents being reviewed, there would be no doubt that an EHCP was necessary.

This is where the homework and long hours came in. I strongly believe that if you sit back at this stage and let the LA do all the work then you are jeopardising the chances of obtaining a robust EHC plan. There is a strict time limit of six weeks for all professionals to send their submissions to the LA. We had six weeks to make sure we contacted all the professionals that could contribute to the assessment process. We also found out that the definition of "consulting" is very loosely interpreted by the LA. Any agency they agreed to consult outside of their own direct resources (such as the NHS) was sent a letter simply asking them if they had anything to contribute to the EHCP assessment process. The routine answer from the agencies seemed to be that "they had nothing to add to the process" and that was the consultation over! We therefore found ourselves having to approach these agencies again and ask for reports or letters that supported our case for an EHCP.

I thought that it would be beneficial for Fraser to see the Speech and Language Therapist (SLT) as part of the process. Fraser had received an SLT assessment and report back in year one, which was very helpful and included a lot about social interaction. As the LA hadn't mentioned they would be asking for a newer one, I figured I should make a parental request. I got on the phone that afternoon to find out what I needed to do to obtain one.

Nothing is ever easy. I called the doctors and spoke to a lady who told me that we wouldn't get an appointment in the timescale that we needed. I explained that this was an emergency, it was for an EHCP assessment and it must be completed. She then paused and mentioned that I could complete a parental referral form but she was unsure if we would get an appointment. What did I have to lose? I wrote all over the form that it was needed for an EHCP assessment and was required ASAP! The same thing happened with CAMHS; I needed to speak to the psychologist that helped diagnose Fraser with Asperger's. I needed to ask for his advice and if he supported a specialist school environment. Getting in touch was much harder than expected! I must have called CAMHS on most days for about three weeks. Each time, I kept getting told he was out of the office or busy. I managed to obtain his email address and again sent him weekly emails about the timeframe we were working to and the valuable input we needed. Then after three weeks, I got a call… it was Ted, the psychologist who assessed Fraser. I was surprised to finally receive a call but felt a sense of relief that finally my communications had been responded to. He sounded unsure as to what I actually needed from him. I explained that all I wanted was a quick email or anything in document form to explain the reasons why Fraser would benefit from being in a specialist setting. He seemed happy enough to help and promised us something via email ... then straight away... there it was!

Just as the email from CAMHS came in, the next email came in from the SLT team. A lovely lady, kind and caring, emailed me offering me an appointment. She mentioned that she could do an observation at the doctor's surgery or at school? I mentioned that school would seem to be the best place as this is where most of the problems were and where Fraser's anxiety was at the worst. She agreed, and booked a date to go visit Fraser in his mainstream school setting. The SLT lady was amazing and very supportive by asking us what we thought would be best for Fraser and keeping in touch with me via email for a few weeks before writing her wonderful report.

Lastly, Nigel and I were concerned that no one was exploring or even acknowledging Fraser's PDA profile. No one wanted, or seemed to want, to put the words in a report because so many different counties were not recognising PDA as a condition. However, the PDA strategies really worked for Fraser, so we felt that if he went to a specialist school that didn't have experience of PDA or even acknowledge it then things would just be the same as mainstream. For this reason, we decided to research what it would take to get a private diagnosis. The only problem here was the cost. We could go private for the diagnosis but knew that private reports would be expensive. Nigel agreed that we needed this in Fraser's EHCP and that we should pursue a diagnosis report as part of the assessment - it was important for us. We booked in to see a private educational psychologist that had been recommended to us in Sheffield. He seemed the most reasonable in cost at around £600, which was a lot cheaper than the cost of a solicitor if the LA decided not to issue an EHCP based on a lack of suitable evidence!

Fraser was due in school that day, but school understood the importance of the appointment. I explained to Fraser that the man we were going to see would be just having a chat with him, all about his clever brain and may do a few puzzles again. He was pretty cool about it and happy to go! We took the trip down to Sheffield and before long, pulled up to a beautiful farmhouse to be greeted by the psychologist, a friendly happy man who just seemed to get Fraser the moment he met him. I waited with him for a while and then went to sit in the warm conservatory whilst the psychologist conducted the assessment with Fraser. I sat waiting nervously, hoping that Fraser was complying but also showing his true colours - exactly the same feeling I had when Fraser was having his autism assessment. Before long, I could see Fraser skipping up the cobbled pathway holding a box of eggs which they chose from the chickens. The man smiled and explained that Fraser has the potential to do amazing - he just needs the right environment - and he would be in touch with his report shortly. A week later, his report landed and I must say it was the most detailed report yet, explaining Fraser to a tee! If half of this information could be incorporated into the assessment and eventually, the final EHCP then we would have the good strong EHCP that Fraser deserved.

I wasn't giving up there though! Next, I wanted an occupational therapist report. Yet again, I was told we had no chance in the time frame requested. However, being polite yet to the point, we managed to get through to the lady that Fraser had seen previously at the doctors. She wrote a report for us all about Fraser's sensory profile. Perfect!

In the meantime, the LA had organised for their own educational psychologist (EP) to attend Fraser's school and hold an observation in class. The EP also met with us and before he wrote his report, I remember thinking that I would be glad when these observations were over. When the EP met with Fraser, I could see Fraser grabbing his cheeks when the EP spoke to him. It was more formal than the private EP we had visited on his farm. I could tell that Fraser was nervous and didn't like the interaction and it was becoming a lot for him to take. He wasn't comfortable, and it was so obvious to see.

Over those six weeks, we collated our reports and evidence and the LA collated theirs. We submitted everything to them and then waited to find out whether, based on an assessment of all this data, the LA would decide whether they thought Fraser needed an EHCP or not. At this stage, we were in constant contact with the caseworker that had been assigned to us. He was a nice man who had recently joined the LA after spending time working in prisons.

He seemed to understand us and we seemed to be trying to achieve the same thing for Fraser – most of the time at least! What echoed in my head during these days was all the warnings I had received from other parents, particularly on the Facebook groups, about how the LA would make us fight for what we wanted, and how bad their experiences were. I hardly ever heard any positive talk about the LA. I always said Facebook helped me - especially the groups I joined. However, at this point, it was causing me more anxiety. The more I read about how others struggled, how others would go to tribunal, the fear was building up inside me. There was a certain level of paranoia that the LA would use tricks to avoid issuing an EHCP or avoid sending children to the right kind of specialist provision. In contrast though, we weren't experiencing any of this.

However – and I think this is a really important point - we never stopped questioning anything we didn't agree with or didn't understand. We spent hours researching the law around the EHCP process, and Nigel even took a two-hour trip to Newcastle to attend a training course run by IPSEA on the legal aspects of obtaining an EHCP. If the LA said or did anything we considered not to be strictly "by the book", we would challenge them. For example, we knew as parents we had a legal right to request the LA properly consult any professional as part of the EHCP assessment process. When we felt the LA were not fulfilling their duty on this point, we called them out on it. We sent an email raising our concern and reminded them of the relevant section in the Children and Families Act. We were never abrupt, rude or demanding. If anything, we were pleasant but very matter of fact and very, very persistent. If our caseworker made a promise to call us but then didn't, we would immediately highlight this. We were also very quick to respond to emails and phone calls. We needed to let the LA know that we were all over the EHCP assessment process and were taking it very seriously. The LA have a mountain of work to deal with, but we were determined that we weren't going to be ignored or treated as "pushover" parents. I truly believe that everyone has to pick their battles and I knew that if the LA were to pick a battle with us, they were going to be in for a very time-consuming slog of it! We had to show them that we were clued up and willing to work hard to ensure our child got the support he so desperately needed.

It wasn't long after submitting our evidence as part of the EHCP assessment process that we received the fantastic news. The LA had assessed everything and decided that they would issue Fraser with an EHCP! This was amazing – from being told that we would never be able to get an EHCP to being granted one was a defining moment for us. The process wasn't over though. We now had the tricky task of agreeing on the contents of the EHCP with the LA and this was absolutely critical as it would determine the type of specialist provision (school) our boy would eventually go to.

We got in touch with our caseworker and asked him what the next steps were. He advised us that first, we would receive a draft EHCP, and then we would be invited to school for a "next steps" meeting to discuss the draft in more detail.

Before long, an email came through with the draft EHCP and we read it in fine detail. The draft was ok to some extent, but we believed it needed a lot of changes. It's important with an EHCP to make sure that it is as specific as possible. This is particularly important in section B and section F of the EHCP.

Section B of an EHCP details the exact special educational needs of the child identified during the assessment process. Section F leads on from this and will contain all the measures that need to be put in place to meet the needs in section B. Both of these sections are known as the "legal" parts of the EHCP, as together they detail what the LA needs to provide for the child by law. The provision set out in the EHCP must be specific with the right level of detail. In addition, it should be quantified. For example, the type of provision along with the hours and frequency of support and level of expertise (Paragraph 9.69 of the Code) needs to be clear. When reading section F of the EHC plan, it should be easy to see the "who, what, when and how long" in relation to each part of the special educational provision.

Our draft EHCP was very general in some areas and didn't quantify how Fraser's needs would be met. We needed specifics. For example, section F contained a line about class sizes and said that they "needed to be small". We had to question what "small" meant though. Did that mean five children or twenty? It was important that these things were nailed down so that there could be no ambiguity that was open to interpretation. Night after late night, Nigel and I sat at the dining room table going through the draft EHCP with a fine toothcomb. Hours and hours we poured into amendments and identifying queries. During this stage, we used the track changes feature in Microsoft Word that showed clearly where we had added, amended or deleted things. This was important so that we could see at a glance where we had requested changes and what kind of change they were. Likewise, when the LA sent us updated versions of the draft we needed to compare the changes they had made to the original document we had sent them. It was important that any deletions or additions were easily identified so we didn't miss anything. Microsoft Word can do this too but there are also free tools available online that are just as good. Solicitors use this kind of method when working on large legal documents and that is exactly what we felt like we were doing. Working on a significant legal document that would shape our child's future.

Eventually, the day of the next steps meeting came. This is a meeting that the current school SENCO, parents, and representatives from the local authority attend. The caseworker commented that our meeting had one of the largest attendances of professionals he had known. On the local authority side was our caseworker, their educational psychologist, the caseworker from the autism specialist unit and the head of the autism specialist unit. We had also invited the lady from SCOPE who had been assisting us throughout this process. We felt it was a good idea to have an outsider's ears to make notes on things we may miss and support us. There were eight people crammed into the small headteacher's office at the school. The next steps meeting should normally run from anything between an hour to two hours. Ours lasted 4 hours with the educational psychologist having to leave for another appointment in the middle of it, followed shortly by the autism specialists.

During the meeting, there seemed to be a reluctance to formally acknowledge our PDA diagnosis. The LA preferred to call it an "opinion".

We pushed back hard on this, Nigel questioned what the difference between a diagnosis and an opinion was? The LA was quick to point out that only recognised conditions could receive a diagnosis and that they didn't recognise PDA formally as a condition. I have got to say, we seemed to go back and forth with this one, arguing that we had received a diagnosis and that it should be acknowledged as such. We eventually agreed to ask the private educational psychologist to change the wording of his report slightly so that we could include a reference to PDA in the final EHCP.

On and on we went, going through the changes we had requested in fine detail. Some of these the caseworker seemed happy to change but others they would not move on. Defining class sizes was a real sticking point. We were eager to ensure that class sizes were no more than six pupils. The caseworker was adamant they couldn't agree to this change. He made the point that finding a school with that kind of class size would be impossible. We argued it wasn't but by the end of the meeting this was a point that for now, we had "agreed to disagree on".

There were quick discussions about the type of setting that they all thought would suit Fraser the best. Our caseworker said that the setting should be calm for Fraser and he agreed that it was best to rule out settings with children who had Social, Emotional and Mental Health (SEMH) issues. Fraser needed to be around children with a profile just like his, and the potential to thrive academically. We knew, however, that there were no settings like this in our local authority area. The LA asked us if we thought that a specialist inclusive learning centre would be a good idea, but again it was a no from us. He would have to access some mainstream schooling for this, and we knew mainstream wasn't going to work. The whole prospect of a mainstream environment, with the rules, discipline, and the way in which pupils needed to conform just wasn't going to work with Fraser. There was no way I was forcing him back into a setting which would cause him to shut down completely.

The school he attended needed to have children just like him. The right school needed to be small and be able to forgive Fraser when he was having trouble with a situation. It needed to have a fun way of learning, with large outdoor spaces for Fraser to run around openly when in meltdown. Fraser has never been a "runner" and is not the type of child that would run away, but with some space to cool down, he is then ready to come back and try again after a short while.

During our meeting, the room fell silent when I mentioned the type of setting we needed. I explained to everyone that the setting we had found would be perfect for Fraser but it was an independent school outside the local authority area. However, our caseworker was at pains to point out that the entry age was nine years old and with Fraser having just turned eight, the age barrier meant that it couldn't be considered at this stage. We mentioned that we would search and look around for an alternate provision and let them know if we find something.

In the meantime, we were informed that as no specialist provision had yet been identified, the final EHCP would have the current (mainstream) school named as the provision in section I, followed by the words "with a move to a specialist provision" at the end. This left us a little uncomfortable as we didn't know legally where this left us. The final EHCP had to be completed within a specific timeframe and we were worried in case we would be stuck with his mainstream setting if an alternative wasn't found soon. The process as a whole is difficult to understand and being able to trust people to do the right thing can be challenging.

Chapter 16 – The Waiting Game

Immediately after the next steps meeting, life continued as normal. Monday morning came around fast, though this morning felt different. Fraser was eating his breakfast, but I could see a glistening in his eyes – he was crying though really trying to hold it in. He was complaining that he felt sick, which wasn't uncommon when he was feeling an extreme level of anxiety. He was worried about going to school. I kept asking myself why I was sending my child to a place that could no longer see to his needs? Fraser wasn't achieving a huge amount at school - he was completely refusing to do most work, and the only work he did was by himself. The rest of the time spent at school was causing Fraser to have high anxiety. Just walking through the school gates over the last few weeks, I could see Fraser's colour drain. I could see he was tired and there was no doubt that this was causing him to feel physically and emotionally tired.

That morning, I made the decision to keep him off school. I wondered why I was sending my child to a setting that was making him feel so poorly and sad? I told Fraser that he could stay off today and I understood why he felt sick. No sooner were the words out of my mouth he flung his arms around me and hugged me tightly. I will give the child credit - he never refused to go to school or got angry with me for taking him. I guess he saw his childhood as very black and white and the rules are that every child has to go to school. However, there must have been some turmoil he wasn't expressing or didn't know how to express. He just wanted to be happy and have friends. However, school was a place where he knew that this could never happen. Not at that time.

That evening when Nigel got home, I explained how exhausted Fraser looked and how I was very worried about how poorly this was making him feel. I didn't want Fraser to go to a school which was causing his anxiety levels to reach a stage that caused him to feel physically sick. I suggested that we may want to keep Fraser off school for his own wellbeing. Nigel was concerned. Nigel has a background working in the legal sector (though wasn't a solicitor), so *he* then started to become anxious about school fines, our obligations as parents and what problems this may cause. At this point, I raised my voice – "let's forget about what the law says - this is our child's health and at the moment his health is deteriorating, and his school have openly said that they can't manage him". Nigel agreed: "Ok – let's go and see the doctor. Let's at least ask their opinion and maybe they can sign him off sick the same as we would if we were feeling depressed or anxious?"

The next day I called the surgery to ask to speak to the doctor. The receptionist advised that we must go in and see them but that we should also take Fraser along. I wasn't too happy that I needed to drag Fraser through yet another meeting about him. I was concerned that he had heard too much negativity in these meetings. He had faced being in the middle of so many after school meetings that I reached the point where I refused to talk to teachers with Fraser also present. This type of communication was damaging to Fraser's self-esteem, and when he was at his lowest, I was hoping the doctor wouldn't need to talk in front of him.

Luckily, we had a nice doctor who completely understood our concerns. He explained that because Fraser is a child, no doctor could sign Fraser off sick - but he would write a letter to school and refer us back to CAMHS due to the level of anxiety that Fraser was facing. The doctor explained that as parents, it is up to us whether Fraser is fit and well enough to go to school or not. Of course, Nigel looked up the law on this one! Nigel mentioned that we must email school weekly and keep them in the loop on Fraser's progress. He also suggested that we ask the school to apply for a resource that specialises in education for children who couldn't attend school due to a medical condition. In my mind, I had already made the decision he wasn't going back the day they said they couldn't meet his needs. That was enough for me. Fraser's anxiety wouldn't be lowered by having a week off, he needed a different setting, and my intention was to have Fraser at home to keep his anxiety at bay until we found another setting that was suitable.

Chapter 17 – Life comes to a Halt

Everything seemed to happen fast. I enjoyed walking the dog and hitting the gym, but now, with Fraser home every day the gym had to come to an end and I cancelled my membership. I had felt that the only time I could have a bit of headspace was when I was at the gym. My gym friends were my main social network and it seemed like I was cutting out a huge part of my life. However, my child needed me now and the right thing to do was give him my 100%. Dog walking was becoming tricky. Fraser wasn't the quickest walker and every walk was hard with a lot of moaning. If it was raining we still had to take the dog out, but Fraser would be walking behind me looking down at the ground, slowly kicking his feet into each puddle that he came in contact with, with me a few steps in front trying to persuade him to walk a little quicker.

With Fraser home full time, things weren't going to be easy until we found a placement, but it was just something we were all going to have to get used to. I told myself it was temporary and that things would go back to normal once again.

I really take my hat off to parents that home school, they do an amazing job. During this time period, we met many parents home-schooling their children, and the parents work around the clock giving their child 100%, with no "me" time. I would read comments on Facebook when half-term was coming up. Parents with children in school would make jokes about how difficult the half term week would be for them. I rolled my eyes and mused about their situation and mine. Whilst there are many of us who are forced into home-schooling, there are also huge numbers who actively choose to home educate as a lifestyle choice. I have friends in both camps. It is rewarding and there are benefits but by god - it's hard work.

My main concern was to ensure Fraser was feeling happy once again, to boost his confidence, and to work with him around his feelings and emotions - which is always tricky for an ASD child. We needed to forget about school for a bit; the pair of us had to, for both our sanity. The thought of not knowing when Fraser would return to a setting that was right for him was a hard thought, and it made me feel very anxious. I would focus all my energy on Fraser, but then I still had the ongoing pressure of finding the right setting for him. I actually started to think that it may be just as easy for me to try and educate Fraser at home. I thought then all the stress would go away, we wouldn't have to go through finding the setting, and I would then have a plan. I would know what was happening.

Not knowing what the future held was the hardest thing, worrying that Fraser would be placed in a setting that wasn't right for him. I worried how long it would take before we found the right setting? What if there were no schools? After all, there is no perfect school - all schools have their advantages and disadvantages, and it was becoming an easier option to home educate. I asked Fraser for his thoughts on staying at home. "We could join home ed groups, Fraser, we don't have to do the normal staying behind a desk all the time. We could go visit places and travel". The options were endless. Fraser looked at me with his big brown eyes "I don't want to do that mummy, I want to go to a school like other children, I want to belong to a school". I understood and had to find the energy to find Fraser a school. I had to find the energy to make this time whilst Fraser was at home fun and bring my happy boy back again. I needed to make him feel wanted and accepted.

The whole process was and is draining when finding the right setting. When, years earlier, I had been finding my eldest sons school placement I had thought that was hard - he had no special needs, and looking back, that was a breeze. This time it was finding a setting where my child would feel accepted, adults who accepted and liked him, who don't use an authoritative approach and have the ability to find it within themselves to wipe the slate clean multiple times a day.

The anticipation of not knowing where my child would belong made my own anxiety high. It was hard each day to try and act "normal," like things were fine, reassuring Fraser that things were ok and putting "the ok face on", but inside I was filled with such worry. Without being able to work off my stress at the gym and feeling like we were in a bit of a rut, I started to feel low on energy. I started to have a few glasses of wine each night to try and forget about my worries and sleep well. However, when you drink more, sleep then turns to disturbed sleep. I was waking in the night swigging on a bottle of Gaviscon from the bedside table as my eating habits had got worse. My bedside table consisted of paracetamols, a large bottle of water and a bottle of Gaviscon. The bedside table stayed like that for a while, I had lost control of me. I no longer felt there was a me and every thought I had was around Fraser and his future.

Every spare minute of the day, I seemed to be checking my emails, anxious in case his current school or the LA were going to start demanding that Fraser returned to school. If I wasn't checking my emails I was engaging with Fraser, trying to work with him. It got to dinner time, Nigel walked through the door, and I would suggest going out to eat. This became an easy option as I didn't feel like cooking anymore. It was easy to go for a bite out, no mess! This happened two to three times a week, drinking a glass or two of wine, having nibbles such as bread and chips, then home for a takeaway. This habit went on for a while; we felt the time away from the house did us good, even if it was just an hour. But as you can imagine that habit wasn't the healthiest and it made me feel even more sluggish. I fell into a lethargic hole, no exercise or social life. There was no me left … I no longer wanted to go out and was happy staying at home with Fraser, it was our safe place. Family wanted to visit but I didn't want to talk. I felt if I opened up to anyone totally, I would just burst in tears, and it was easier to hide behind my phone or the keyboard and tell people that all was fine. In reality, I was anxious and worried and sometimes, even scared at what the future held. Nigel would hold me tight and reassure me that everything would work out in the end. He told me lots of times -

what is the worst that can happen? Fraser stays at home and we try and find the money for tutors - even though I knew this would mean no family holidays or spare money, as it would all be thrown into giving Fraser some kind of education. Nigel was the only one holding me together at this point. I had to trust him that things would work out fine and to stop worrying myself. Generally, when Nigel tells me something will be fine, it normally is so I had to trust him on this but naturally I couldn't help but worry. I've got to say it's the worst feeling in the world knowing that these professionals would decide on my child's school and I was so worried that I wouldn't really have a say in it. What if I found a setting and had to fight the LA for it? There were plenty of "what ifs".

Nigel and I needed a day/night away for a bit of time together. All our spare time was taken with talking about the situation, his EHCP, the right setting, and what the future held for Fraser. We were both drained but needed some time to think. Fraser was constantly under our feet and he was hearing us talk about all of this. He was fed up of listening about his parents' worry and concern, and it wasn't good for him to hear our discussions. He even brought it to our attention one night whilst we were sat having a takeaway - how he was trying to get our attention but all we ever did was talk about the EHCP. Fraser knew that we were doing this for him, but at the same time he was fed up of the process as much as we were.

However, there was no escape from the EHCP process and we needed to look at the draft that we had in front of us without Fraser listening. We had to ensure that the LA did not try to push a mainstream setting on us and checking the draft version of the EHCP was critical to ensure this couldn't happen. We knew that mainstream wasn't going to work - we had tried it for four years, alongside every strategy that his mainstream school could offer.

Money was tight, and we were worried in case we needed to go to tribunal and had to pay for a solicitor. We couldn't afford a fancy night away - so mum offered to let us stay at her flat for the evening. She would come to ours and sit with Fraser. That way, we had the added bonus of not being too far away in case Fraser became difficult and we needed to go back home, so we took my mum up on her offer. We decided to go to a hotel in Harrogate during the day to focus on reviewing the draft EHCP. It would be quiet, we could have lunch there, a few drinks and take the laptop! We could go through the draft EHCP in fine detail and add our comments by the deadline, and then use the rest of the day to relax once that was done. Some people may have thought we were crazy for not using the opportunity to completely switch off – given everything that was going on around us. We couldn't rest though. We knew it needed doing, and if we could do it without Fraser being able to hear, then it was a good time to really concentrate with no disturbances. We spent most of the afternoon at the hotel and really pulled the EHCP apart and wrote all our reasons why a mainstream setting wasn't going to be right for Fraser. After four hours we were burnt out. We had a nice meal and then went back to my mum's. Our plan had been to get changed and go for a couple of drinks locally. Instead of going out, we ended up falling asleep fully clothed on the bed exhausted, and woke up the next morning having slept through completely!

Chapter 18 - A New Setting

One thing that stuck in my mind from the next steps meeting, was the SENCO looking nervously at the draft EHCP and explaining to the caseworker her worry that the school simply couldn't meet Fraser's needs detailed in there. She had been very supportive throughout the process whilst we were trying to find another school that could meet Fraser's needs. However, she was obviously worried in case the LA expected her school to try and meet all of Fraser's needs. The sad story was that there was no school that would be able to do this in our area.

There are some amazing schools in our area for children with more extreme disabilities but whilst Fraser had some complex requirements, he didn't have the same type of disabilities or challenges as the children in the schools we had toured. With a PDA diagnosis as part of his ASD, he was bright but hard to teach and engage. I started my research into out of authority specialist schools that were no more than a one hour drive away. Once again, I turned to the Facebook groups to see if anyone could offer a recommendation. I had made friends with one lady in particular, who said that Fraser reminded her of her son. At the time, she was fighting for the same school that we had wanted to send Fraser to, only to be thwarted by the entry age. Whilst I was chatting to her on Facebook Messenger, she mentioned another school that she had viewed over the opposite side of Yorkshire. It was a forty-five-minute drive from us and she was very impressed with how the adults approached the students when she went to visit. The only worry she had was that a majority of the children had SEMH (Social, Emotional and Mental Health) issues. Nevertheless, I needed to go and see for myself – what did I have to lose?

I picked up the phone excitedly to arrange an appointment! The lady on the phone was keen for us to come and visit, and arranged for me to attend in the next couple of days. I started to feel excited, we may have found the right school!

The school is for children across a broad spectrum of needs - including social, emotional and mental health, ADHD (Attention Deficit/Hyperactivity Disorder), PDA, Autism and attachment disorder. I was advised from groups on Facebook that SEMH children and Asperger's children may not mix well as the Asperger's children may need a quieter and calmer environment. However, I thought I would keep our options open and visit the school anyhow. Fraser was no angel in the classroom and would lash out at others, so a tiny part of me thought a setting such as this may help with his social and emotional problems.

The date came, it was summer and we were experiencing a heatwave. I remember driving down the long narrow road that led to the main school building and looking at all the fields that surrounded it. The school was in a remote area out of the way. It had a calm feel to it and was extremely quiet. I had a tour of the school and was blown away. There were therapy houses to provide art therapy, drama therapy, music therapy, a cinema room, an art room, a design and a technology room with machines that Fraser would be allowed to use. There was den building and forest school once a week, and importantly - small class sizes. It all seemed too good to be true - how amazing! I had to ask the question "Is it hard for the LA to give such a place to a child? I am guessing it's an expensive placement for the LA?" The lady who was showing me around looked at me and said if you think it's the right school then all I will say is fight for it.

I walked away, knowing that this felt like the right place. We needed to ask for this school, but it might be a fight - we knew that the fees were high due to it being an independent school. Would we get it, who knows? We could but try! That evening, we emailed our caseworker to let him know that we had found a school that we believed was capable of meeting Fraser's needs. So far, the LA hadn't come up with anything in our local area. Fraser was complex with PDA and ASD but able to achieve. He was a bright boy with a bright future ahead so long as he was in the right setting.

The LA would have to go through a process to determine whether they were prepared to fund Fraser's place there. First of all, the school would have to confirm that they could meet Fraser's needs. They reviewed his draft EHCP and quickly confirmed that they could meet his needs and had a place available for him. However, as the school fees were high, the LA needed to go to an internal panel which takes place on a Thursday. We would wait for an outcome and the decision would come from a senior manager. Everything seemed to drag, but there was a process that had to be followed and Nigel reminded me that I must be patient and remain calm. I could feel it in my bones that something would get in our way – we would be turned down and I might need to put our boxing gloves back on. I braced myself for a fight.

A few days later, my phone started ringing. I had just come back from walking the dog. It was a nice warm afternoon and I was in my own little bubble, pacing down the street towards home. Nigel was on the other end of the phone: "Katie, I have just spoken with the caseworker - we have got the placement at the school! It's the nearest school that can meet needs and we have got Fraser a start date in September".

"What?!!", I retorted. "You must be joking right? No fight? No questions? We've just got it?" I think I asked Nigel the same question over and over again "What the hell?" "How?!!"

Excitement ran through my body and at the same time a huge weight lifted off my shoulders. I can't explain the number of emotions that I was feeling right then! I couldn't believe it - all my worries over with and things were going to be back to normality. I walked through the door and shouted to Fraser. I said to him "We have something really great to tell you Fraser! You know the school with the farm and the small class sizes and the people that understand you … well you have a place and you're going to be starting in September! How amazing is that!" Fraser jumped up and down with excitement. He was so happy, as much as we were! I held him so tightly and told him that this was his new start and it was going to be amazing. Fraser was looking forward to going to view the school.

My next thought was to call my mum. My mum is my best friend and she knew how hard things were for Fraser, she had been an ear to listen to me from day one. My mum herself struggled with Fraser and knew he needed this help and support. I called her and screamed, "He has a place mum, he has got it!" Mum was as excited as all of us. We were all happy - the whole family was affected by Fraser's behaviours and every one of us at times had been reduced to tears, only because we all love Fraser so much. We just wished for him to be happy and understood.

The head of his new school was just as surprised as we were; he couldn't believe that the council had agreed to the placement so quickly but seemed very happy that things were running fast and smoothly. We asked when Fraser would be able to visit the school. He replied that we would be allowed to visit as soon as we liked, but the other boys wouldn't be present as they were out on day trips as it was the last week before the summer holidays! I explained that I thought it would be a good idea to show Fraser the school even if the children weren't present. I needed to make sure that Fraser had seen his school otherwise the summer holidays would be filled with anxiety not knowing what to expect.

The day for the visit came, the sun was blazing and a warm gentle breeze in the air. We rolled up to the school and Fraser was expectant about what was to come. A nice down to earth lady met us and arranged to show us around. The school was quiet but Fraser was happy to be shown around, we went into a few rooms but the alarm went off because they had been locked. I was starting to panic as I knew Fraser wouldn't like the loud noise but he seemed to cope. We managed to do the tour and despite the alarms going off he was excited to start his new journey.

Starting a New School

We had visited the school at the start of the summer holidays so there was a few weeks wait before Fraser could start. The weeks passed quickly though and before we knew it the start date came around. On the first day at his new school, we were all nervous and unsure of what to expect. I was hoping that Fraser wouldn't lash out at any pupils or staff. I was keeping everything crossed! Fraser was given the choice to do part of the week rather than a full week, as he had been off school for some time now. I asked him what he would prefer to do; he said he must go straight away and do a full week. His logic was, if he went part-time and struggled with change, he didn't want to use that as an excuse not to go. He thought it would be best to crack on with a full week so he didn't have to go through a longer and more gradual change, which he would struggle with more. I could completely understand Fraser's logic behind this, and I must say I was super proud of his positive attitude.

School starts late morning on a Monday, so we had a shorter day to break the ice. Fraser entered the classroom where the class was in the middle of a baking lesson. Immediately, Fraser piped up: "Baking is rubbish!" Fraser has always enjoyed baking, but immediately he was testing the water and wanting to know how the teachers would respond. Would they shout at him? Would they tell him to leave the classroom? Would they restrain him? The teacher running the class quickly responded, "Fine Fraser, we have other things you may want to do? How about some maths?" Fraser started shouting at the top of his voice: "boring boring boring - I am not doing anything!" The teacher was going to experience Fraser's demand avoidance pretty quick! He came up to Fraser and pointed towards a table and chair in the corner of the class, with this Fraser lost it and kicked him. The teacher ignored this behaviour and passed him over to his key worker to calm down. That day when I collected him he ran into my car and burst into tears. "Oh no Fraser, what on earth has happened?" He replied, "I didn't make any biscuits, everyone else was allowed to take biscuits home and I have none". I felt a lump in my throat. All I wished for was his first day to be positive, but then I figured that it may be tricky and things would get better. I held the tears back to remain strong for Fraser, and we drove home hoping that the next day would be better.

Fraser learnt the harsh way that if he refused to take part, the consequence was - no biscuits to take home. Fraser cried about how one of the teachers had grabbed his arm; he said that he had dragged him out of the class. I figured Fraser may have become confused between restraints and, possibly, him just being sensitive to others touching him. In the back of my head I did question why there had been a physical intervention so quickly but I also knew that when Fraser kicked out, he should be prevented from hurting others. All I wanted was a good day…maybe I was asking too much.

The next day when we rolled up to school, both of us were in a positive frame of mind. Fraser still complained about being taken from class the previous day and I was concerned that this was going to bother him going forward. I needed to mention this to the staff as we needed Fraser to trust them. If he couldn't trust staff from the outset, we were heading for a bad start. The next day flew by. I was constantly checking my phone waiting for it to ring but I heard nothing. I wish I had been a fly on the wall. It wasn't fair; I guess no news was good news? 3.30pm couldn't come fast enough and I was dying to find out how Fraser's day had gone. I was sitting alone in the car outside his school when out of nowhere, the back door opened and Fraser threw himself into the car. His eyes filled up with tears and my heart sank. "What's happened now darling?" He blurted, "I was told to eat with my knife and fork - they told me off because I ate my chips with my fingers, so I ran out of the dining hall". I rolled my eyes without Fraser seeing and thought I must make an appointment to see the headteacher. Fraser's EHCP mentioned that he struggled with a knife and fork and would need extra help from the occupational therapist with this. I started to feel concerned that all our effort and work for the EHCP was being ignored so early on. I was feeling deflated because I thought that Fraser was doing amazing with the change. He wasn't used to having a cooked dinner at school; we used to stick with packed lunches, so Fraser knew what he was going to eat. To keep anxiety at a low level, I would give him the choice of what he would like to eat in his packed lunch. Eating a school dinner was a big enough step. I asked the headteacher why he was pulled up at lunch about his knife and fork and explained that I thought it was trivial to be so picky this early on. He then explained that they had Fraser's best interests at heart. They didn't want him to be bullied by other boys because he was throwing sweetcorn and peas from the palm of his hand into his mouth. Again, I thought maybe I was just being the overprotective mum? I have fought his corner for such a long time. When do you ever stop fighting your child's corner, hey? I'm currently still doing it. It's never going to stop.

There were some additional incidents that troubled us. On one day, just after starting, Fraser had been pushed to the ground. In a separate incident Fraser had been thrown into the railings in the playground, and then there seemed to be a general theme of the older boys calling Fraser "midget". I tried to explain to Fraser that it would be a bit odd if he was taller than them considering he was the youngest boy in the school! If anything, this was a huge learning curve for Fraser.

At his new school, he had finally seen other boys angry and frustrated – and oddly, this made him start to realise that sometimes others struggle too. It wasn't just him that had difficulties. Despite some initial hiccups; he really found himself in those early few weeks. Fraser's confidence boomed, my happy boy was back again. Something clicked into my beautiful boy's head. For so long, he had felt like the only angry, naughty boy. Children had sniggered and pointed at him, he was restrained regularly, and all this was behind him. At his new school, he finally realised that he wasn't the only boy that felt like this. He no longer felt different as he was in a school where all the boys were going through their own struggles. Furthermore, he started to reflect on how his behaviour at his previous school had impacted his classmates. Fraser's smile came back, Fraser started to feel compassionate about others and wanted to help others around him become happy again, just like he was feeling right now. I always worried about Fraser's compassion for others, but it was shining out of him like a flower blooming, for the first time.

There were boys that Fraser had run-ins with, but things always worked out. Fraser said he was scared of them but he felt that they would become friends eventually. Call it a sixth sense, he was right - they are friends now. Fraser listened to me when I explained that other boys in the school might not be friendly straight away. They may have felt a huge sense of rejection for longer than Fraser, and the only way they knew how to respond was through their fight mode. I promised Fraser that baby steps would eventually form a friendship, and I was right. All it takes for most of these kids is to feel accepted; once they feel safe and accepted, they can flourish.

Fraser was flying, he was moved up a class with older boys within the first month and was learning again. He was writing and joining in with activities. There were minor issues, but when I compared them to the positives, I was pretty happy. We had seen a huge amount of change in Fraser; his confidence was back and he no longer felt like his learning was at a disadvantage. Fraser is a bright boy, but due to something called "delayed processing", which is part of his autism, it took him a little longer than others to understand instructions. Once he understood though, he was motivated and loved doing his work. Fraser started to ask for homework as he wanted to do a qualification in information technology. I never thought that my child would ask for homework!

Fraser was engaging in forest school. It was hard enough to get Fraser out on a dog walk so I was really unsure about forest school; but he loved it. He was getting exercise participating in the den building, and learning about different types of trees, plants and materials.

Fraser was also now going into school assemblies. That's one thing he hated at mainstream - entering the assembly hall. He would refuse blankly to enter, secluding himself even more. This time around was different. I heard he was going into assemblies and would immediately raise his hand to speak out loud to show others how much he knew about a subject, or to answer a question. He read out loud to all seventy pupils, the teachers sitting there, with their mouths on the floor. Fraser was the youngest child but was becoming an articulate and confident reader there. The staff would tell me how proud they felt that they had a child as young as Fraser who could read as well as he could.

This next one shocked me. On collection one day, I was told that Fraser had been involved in a swimming gala. We had always paid for one to one swimming lessons as Fraser could not bear any other child in his space. Swimming and the pool area would cause Fraser to shut down and go under the water to get away from being overloaded with the loudness of the pool, the other children and the commotion. To hear that he took part in a gala was just outstanding! Fraser's teacher that evening messaged me to let me know how pleased he was that

Fraser had accomplished such an event. Even during one to one swimming lessons, the demands were tricky and swimming was never easy. His PDA took over during these lessons and he needed to be better than anyone else. His confidence was now back, and I believe the one to one lessons had given him a head start compared to others that were older but hadn't been lucky enough to have additional swimming lessons over the last few years. I was told that Fraser wanted to enter every competition at the gala, which he couldn't unfortunately. He understood this but was very keen.

Then came the Christmas concert. Wow - he blew me away. He had a reading piece and read very clearly and was so confident. I nudged the man next to me to tell him that was my son reading! I was so proud, previously he had only got small parts in a play with possibly seven words to remember at a push. This time he was given a poem to read. He was very capable of doing it and I knew there would be no sniggers from parents or other children. We were all in the same boat and everyone understood the battle each boy had with themselves just to get up there, it was a lovely feeling. I did watch him throughout the concert putting his hands to his ears to block out the noise as parents clapped after each carol had been sung. Even though he did well reading in front of so many people, he found the overall experience tricky, but managed to sit through it for over an hour and a half amongst two hundred and fifty people. At the end, he looked pale and worn out. It was too much even though he tried to hold it together and manage. After the concert, there were refreshments for parents, but we decided it was time to escape with our boy, and missed the refreshments. Fraser was complaining that he felt sick, and he really didn't look great. We walked to the car for a deep breath of air. He sat in the back and explained how he had felt so much better now he was out of there. "Two hundred and fifty people mum and dad - that was a lot of people!" he exclaimed seriously. "I think I felt sick because it was too busy". He totally understood himself and was in tune with how he was feeling. He had done amazing and we let him know how super proud we were of him! There was, and is, so many amazing things that have happened in the last three months since Fraser started this school.

The school has an abundance of caring and dedicated staff members and Fraser gets the one to one support he needs on a daily basis. Many of the staff have been there years and their experience in dealing with the challenges faced by the boys is second to none. They identify the positives in each boy and nurture their natural skills and talents to the point where the boys start to feel the things they never did before – self-esteem, confidence and belonging.

Chapter 19 - The Future

It's about six months since I wrote the previous chapters. Fraser's life (and ours) have changed for the better, in ways we wouldn't have believed during some of those darker days.

I wanted to tell you all the positives as I believe this process in Fraser's life has been a life-changer for our little boy. Small steps at a time, and never forgetting to fight your child's corner.

However, despite some great positives in those first few months of his new school, I became worried that it wasn't going to be right for him. To be honest, we nearly took Fraser out of there. On that initial visit, it had seemed perfect but then we had a series of issues that caused us some serious doubt. Is there ever a right setting? I don't think there is a perfect setting, and from experience, Fraser has understood that every child can be different, they face their own battles and may not overcome them as quickly as he has.

Fraser has learnt so much, but he also hasn't faced trauma in his life like some of the children at his school. Fraser sometimes struggles as he perceives some of the other children want to continuously annoy him; he doesn't understand why they don't want to learn like him, and a few times, I have seen him copying behaviours from other children.

There were a few incidents that worried us and we initially had some doubts about the environment. The school has hardworking and dedicated staff but when Fraser came home complaining that he was being picked on from time to time we became concerned. We had a lot of meetings with senior staff who were always there to listen and provide reassurance but it was a delicate time for us. After our experiences with mainstream school we were desperate for everything to go to plan. With a seed of doubt thrown into my mind, I needed to know what my plan B was going to be if this new school didn't work out. So in those early days of his new school, we tried applying again for the school that we had originally hoped for. Fraser was coming up to the right age to go on their waiting list for assessment. I needed to ask our LA if we could move, despite all the positives of his new school he kept telling us that he wasn't happy. In order to consider a change of school once an EHCP is in place, an emergency review of the EHCP must take place. An emergency review was required as part of the process to draft a new EHCP and with that, the naming of a new school.

We had a good conversation with the headteacher at his new school. He was understanding but saddened that we were thinking of a move so quickly. I explained that I was concerned for Fraser and that we understood it was a difficult situation to resolve. The school was for those children that had been refused elsewhere, and the school does a brilliant job in offering acceptance to those children. During that conversation with the head, I waited for my moment to ask a cheeky question; if things didn't work out, or if we decided that we didn't want to move him - could we keep things as they were here? I guess I was pretty confused; it was a hard decision - we rock the boat and move our child that is doing well in so many areas, and things don't work out again! It was a huge risk. The headteacher told me that if at any time we wanted to put a stop to it all we could, and they would happily keep Fraser there. That comforted me somewhat. I was scared and wasn't sure we were doing the right thing.

The day finally came for the emergency review. I stepped out of the car and followed Nigel into the school meeting room a nervous wreck. I began telling myself to keep acting confident and not to worry, but when you're in a room with another nine adults from various professions, it gets scary. We all sat around a table; it was a warm day and the fan was blowing in the corner. Each professional – teachers, therapists and support workers - took it in turns to talk about how well Fraser was doing and what he was achieving. Then it came to us and we were asked the question about why we wanted to move Fraser.

I could feel my hands shaking and a lump in my throat. When it's your son's future and you don't want to mess up it becomes an immense amount of pressure that just keeps building. I spoke about how Fraser felt picked on and he needed a calmer environment. All the faces around me dropped and glared with shock. They told me that they had seen our little boy wandering the grounds, day in, day out with a smile on his face and forming friendships.

They seemed confused that we had a completely different story compared to what they saw every day.

We expressed to the LA caseworker, who was also present at the meeting, that we were encouraged about all the good feedback we had heard and thought the school do an amazing job; however, we were still keen to find an alternative provision. The caseworker from our LA explained that she would consult with the other independent school we had originally seen, however, she must also consult with local schools to see if they could meet Fraser's needs.

I was a little confused - why would she say this - because just under eight months ago, no school in our local area could meet Fraser's needs, unless the LA had built a new school?

We found out that the LA had done just that. They had built a new school, which was an autism hub connected to a large mainstream school. Exactly the type of environment that wasn't right for my boy. I needed to call and speak to the person in charge of the hub to ask some questions. I spoke, and explained that Fraser always longed to be with pupils just like him; since the move to his recent specialist school, he no longer felt different or separated out from others, a unit would only make Fraser feel different again. Fraser would want to be in the mainstream school and he would try to fit in, but sadly couldn't because of his social difficulties and his sensory needs - his whole self-esteem would take a huge tumble, and then you would have the same boy that he was back at mainstream primary - in fight mode. There is no possible way that a unit attached to a mainstream school would work for our child.

Still unsure we were doing the right thing, and

conscious of the risks, we sat down one evening and spoke to Fraser. He was ever so mature for an eight-year-old child, and sometimes his understanding blows me away. We explained that the LA had found another school but it was in a unit attached to a mainstream. Straight away his eyebrows raised, like a little old man's. "There is no way I'm going to that!" We spoke to him about the choices, and he decided he wanted to stay where he was and try things again. He didn't want us to be on the education fight again, and to some degree, it had affected us all as a family the first time around. Collating reports and making the EHCP fit tightly to his needs and the school, it would have to happen all over again.

A part of me was relieved, but then another part of me was sad - have we failed our son? Are we doing the right thing? All I want is for him to be happy, feel safe and feel understood. We advised the school and the LA that Fraser had decided to stay. Everyone seemed very happy that he was going to be there for a while longer yet.

Once the decision was made to stay, that week seemed to be the best week ever; the uncertainty had gone. Fraser started to look happy once again and I wasn't been told a story each night about what had gone wrong in the day. I was actually hearing what was going right!

At first, when Fraser got in the car at 3pm, I daren't ask him if he'd had a good day. I think that, deep down, I didn't want to know in case things were bad so I stayed quiet. However, I didn't need to ask - he would jump in the car with a smile on his face, and that would tell me straight away that things were positive.

4 Months Later

What a difference! Things have really changed - Fraser has found a close circle of friends that are very similar to himself, and he is growing into a happy little boy, which then makes him want to learn - he is flying high. He is a popular boy at school, even the older boys make time for him and give him props.

The school offered him a job as an IT assistant. It has given him a purpose and made him feel important. He's also been chosen to be a digital leader, which will see him go to other schools and homes for the elderly to talk about internet safety - widening his social skills and boosting his confidence even further. He had just returned from a five-day residential trip and loved it. It was a huge worry for me, having him away from the security of the family and everything he knows for a few days. The staff said he was brilliant. Well behaved and a zest for everything they did.

This weekend was an important weekend - he has turned nine years old. We decided to invite a few friends to go to his favourite store, Game and play on the consoles there, followed by McDonalds for lunch, and then a visit to the cinema. Three boys from his school attended, and they were all little gems; the excitement on these kid's faces knowing that they had been invited to a party was priceless.

These children, including Fraser, had been classed as naughty boys previously and wouldn't get party invites in their old school environments. The impact on their self-esteem, by feeling normal, and part of a friendship group is amazing. To just be invited filled them all with joy, and most importantly they felt wanted again.

Fraser had an amazing day, and the most amazing gift that he received this year was friendship. That evening, I looked at my husband with a tear in my eye and said "We've done this! We have got him into the right school, and he's made friends".

The future is bright for Fraser, and I have to say it is all down to the education setting; with the right support and understanding, your child will fly. Never give up. Even in the dark days, something made us carry on through the exhaustion, the negativity, and the never-ending barriers.

If we can do it, you can too.

Katie Stott
July 2019

Abbreviations

One of the biggest challenges for us was dealing with the sheer amount of abbreviations and jargon used by professionals through the autism diagnosis and EHCP process. We have created the table below that will hopefully make things a little easier for you.

Abbreviation	Meaning
ASD	**Autism Spectrum Disorder.** A developmental disorder that is characterized by difficulties in social interaction and communication and by restricted or repetitive patterns of thought and behaviour.
EHCP	**Education Health and Care Plan**. This is a legal document that describes a child or young person's special educational, health and social care needs.
IEP	**Individual Education Plan**. A document that helps teaching staff to plan for a child. It should include strategies to help them learn and be used to review their progress. Very different to an EHCP.
LA	**Local Authority.** Generally used to refer to the education and/or

	children's services department within local government.
PDA	**Pathological Demand Avoidance**. A developmental disorder which is distinct from autism but falls under the spectrum, first identified by Elizabeth Newson in 2003, although it is still not currently recognised in many tools used for diagnosing autism.
SEN	**Special Educational Needs.** Used to describe learning difficulties or disabilities that make it harder for children to learn than most children of the same age. Children with Special Educational Needs are likely to need extra or different help from that given to other children their age.
SENCO	**Special Educational Needs Co-Ordinator.** The school teacher who is responsible for assessing, planning and monitoring the progress of children with special needs.

Assistance

There are several fantastic support groups and organisations that can help families who need to know more about Autism, Asperger's, PDA and the EHCP process. We have detailed them here. All details are correct at the time of going to print.

National Autistic Society

The UK's largest provider of specialist autism services. They have a special autism helpline:

Call: **0808 800 4104**.
Their lines are open 10am-4pm from Monday-Thursday. On Fridays, they are open from 9am-3pm (excluding Bank Holidays).

Website: www.autism.org.uk
Email: nas@nas.org.uk

PDA Society

The PDA Society provide information, support and training for parents, carers, teachers and individuals with PDA. They also work hard to push awareness of PDA.

Enquiries can be submitted via their website. They aim to respond to each enquiry in 3-5 days.

Website: https://www.pdasociety.org.uk
Email: info@pdasociety.org.uk

Facebook Groups

During some of my darkest times the greatest support came from Facebook groups. Here are some of the groups that have helped me reach out to parents and carers facing similar challenges.

Life on an Alien Planet
(**https://www.facebook.com/groups/lifenonanalien planet/**)

My own Facebook group that helps parents and carers of children with forms of Autism and PDA.

The SEND VCB Project
(**https://www.facebook.com/groups/4218392881509 39/**)

This group is run by the amazing Yvonne Newbold. It is for families of children up to the age of 18, who also have a Neuro-Developmental Condition such as Autism, ADHD, PDA or a Learning Disability, and who are violent towards others at home or elsewhere.

PDA Yorkshire
(**https://www.facebook.com/groups/1015873185119 572/**)

Run by my good friend Ruth, this is a Yorkshire-based PDA support group open to parents (and primary caregivers) of children with (suspected) Pathological Demand Avoidance.

Made in the USA
Las Vegas, NV
20 August 2022

53572308R00111